Advance Praise for *Business from Bed*

"No matter where you are in a personal healthcare crisis, *Business from Bed* will empower you to be the ultimate navigator of your journey; rediscover yourself, be inspired and begin to understand it's not who you are or your diagnosis that defines you, but what you do to embrace life and start living."
—**Amy Ohm**, CEO and Co-founder, TreatmentDiaries.com™

"This book is a helpful "companion" if you need to find out how to come back to business after a life-changing event. It provides tools to explore new directions when you are prompted to review your goals, values, and lifestyle because of a health setback."
—**Ilona Rudolfs**, Business Owner in The Netherlands living with UC (ulcerative colitis) and Life Coach for Business Owners Living with Health Setbacks.

"Thank you Joan Friedlander for being a powerful voice to motivate individuals working with health challenges. *Business from Bed*—A MUST HAVE for all life coaches and health care professionals working interdependently with others."
—**Sheila K. Dameron-Dixon**, Founder, Women Building & Investing in Success

"Joan addresses a topic that so many avoid…a topic which is near to my heart. I have been quite ill over my life and this book is a **blueprint for resilience.** Her approach to, not only, physical resilience but mental, emotional and spiritual resilience is spot on!

In 1983 I almost died from a staph infection in my bone, the same year I was detained in E. Africa…so I am impressed with her ability to embrace adversity and make it work for you on your way back to doing business.

Her modalities, such as drawing and visual expression, help people embrace their inner struggles but also create their new 'story' and accept where they have been and who they were meant to become. As a witness to healing, you can in turn become the Healer."
—**Heather P. Shreve**, Certified Wellcoach, Behavior Specialist, Author: *Drawn Into Wellness: Train Your Brain to Create Lasting Change* and *Caught on The Equator: Finding The Fire Within*, Founder: www.lifeguardwellness.com

"Joan Friedlander has written a wonderful gem! *Business from Bed* offers inspiration and practical advice for anyone who experienced a chronic illness and wants to get their life back. I would highly recommend Ms. Friedlander's book for professionals in the health service field or to anyone who works with the chronically ill. Ms. Friedlander offers anyone with a chronic illness wisdom and hope!"
—**Bob Zukowski**, Vocational Rehabilitation Consultant

"Joan provides a comprehensive, yet simple; step by step plan to navigate through a health crisis by integrating both emotional and physical healing. Her approach is practical, kind, and ultimately very human."

—**Dr. Crystal Frazee, PT**, CrystalFrazee.com

"Ironically, I heard about Joan's book in the middle of a health episode. It was my first time having surgery and of course, I was concerned about the continuity of my daily life as I recovered. As a business owner, wife and Mom, my life was hectic. Then everything stopped. Business from Bed is important because it helped me effectively deal my businesses coming to a halt as I recovered. After reading the book I reflected on what aspects of my life should change going forward. I learned to delegate more. I also chose to focus on God, family, friends and good health. Thanks, Joan."

—**Vanessa Maddox**, Founder and Chief Executive Girlfriend, TheGirlfriendGroup

"Business from Bed is the must-have book for anyone challenged by illness, but wants a career! The six steps Joan provides give you what you need to deal with the emotional and psychological burden of illness, design a career that fits your needs while nurturing your soul and tips to be successful."

— **Leslie Truex**, Owner of WorkAtHomeSuccess.com and Author of *The Work-At-Home Success Bible*

"Practical, thoughtful, and insightful. Joan draws on her expertise, compassion, and engaging writing style to create and excellent resource for anyone returning to work after a health crisis."

—**Donna Sales, R. Psych**, Founder of the website Hope Café, www.hopecafe.net

"*Business from Bed* shares many inspiring stories of people with health issues finding creative ways to reinvent their work persona. But it goes much further than just sharing stories. Joan has laid out a step-by-step plan on how to set up a business that deals with your particular health issues. She also deals with how to restore your confidence that you are a just as valuable to your clients now as you were before your health challenges. This book is not just for those with health issues but is equally valuable for anyone who has is faced with a major change in their career. Great coaching, Joan!"

—**Doug Gfeller**, Master Certified Coach

Business from Bed

Business from Bed

The 6-Step Comeback Plan to Get Yourself Working Again After a Health Crisis

Joan Friedlander

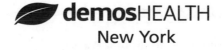

demosHEALTH

New York

Visit our website at www.demoshealth.com

ISBN: 978-1-936303-44-1
e-book ISBN: 978-1-617051-43-2

Acquisitions Editor: Noreen Henson
Compositor: diacriTech

Medical information provided by Demos Health, in the absence of a visit with a health care professional, must be considered as an educational service only. This book is not designed to replace a physician's independent judgment about the appropriateness or risks of a procedure or therapy for a given patient. Our purpose is to provide you with information that will help you make your own health care decisions.

The information and opinions provided here are believed to be accurate and sound, based on the best judgment available to the authors, editors, and publisher, but readers who fail to consult appropriate health authorities assume the risk of injuries. The publisher is not responsible for errors or omissions. The editors and publisher welcome any reader to report to the publisher any discrepancies or inaccuracies noticed.

Library of Congress Cataloging-in-Publication Data

Friedlander, Joan.
  Business from Bed : the 6-step comeback plan to get yourself working again after a health crisis / Joan Friedlander.
     p. cm.
  ISBN 978-1-936303-44-1
  1. Work capacity evaluation. 2. Vocational rehabilitation. 3. Medicine, Industrial. 4. Convalescence. 5. People with disabilities—Employment. 6. Chronically ill—Employment. 7. Businesspeople—Health and hygiene. I. Title.
  RC963.4.F75 2013
  362.16023–dc23

                              2012035142

Special discounts on bulk quantities of Demos Health books are available to corporations, professional associations, pharmaceutical companies, health care organizations, and other qualifying groups. For details, please contact:

Special Sales Department
Demos Medical Publishing, LLC
11 West 42nd Street, 15th Floor
New York, NY 10036
Phone: 800-532-8663 or 212-683-0072
Fax: 212-941-7842
E-mail: rsantana@demosmedpub.com

Printed in the United States of America by Bang Printing.
12 13 14 15 / 5 4 3 2 1

For my son, who lived through it.
To my husband, who supported me and never (rarely)
complained.

In honor of the clients, colleagues, friends, and mentors
who have inspired me without knowing it.

Contents

Foreword

When my friend and colleague Joan Friedlander first suggested to me that *Business from Bed* might be the title of her next book, I laughed delightedly. "It's perfect," I said. I remember all too well how, during a health crisis of my own, I ran my business from bed on many occasions. There I would be, propped up in bed with pillows, wearing PJ's and my telephone headset, notepad and pen in my lap, having sessions with my coaching clients. And never saying a word to my clients about what things were like on my end of the phone.

As the author of the bestselling *Get Clients Now!*, and a business coach who has worked with thousands of entrepreneurs over the past two decades, I'm intimately familiar with the struggle of trying to maintain one's business or career during and after a health crisis. I've helped many of my clients through times like these, and I've been there myself, as you will learn later in this book.

When you are ill or injured, your number one priority has to be your health, and your second priority must often be your family because of the impact your health issues have on them. So your business or job ends up taking a back seat, sometimes for an extended period. But then comes the time when you must return to making a living, and you also crave the satisfaction and self-esteem that comes from performing your chosen work. How do you get back to business?

That's where *Business from Bed* comes in. The comeback plan in this book will help you rise from the ashes of your health crisis in a new form, suited for who and how you are today. You'll learn how to redesign your business or job—or find a new one—that fits what you are able to do, and desire to do most. You'll find strategies, tools, and advice from Joan and others who have walked this road to help you recover, rebuild, and succeed.

Joan is uniquely qualified to write this book. She has the business experience to advise readers about strategizing, organizing, managing, and finances. She has the coaching experience needed to provide smart questions, helpful structures, perspective, and encouragement. And she has years of personal experience to share about her own battles with chronic illness.

I first met Joan in 2001. She was referred to me by another coach—Joan and I both have long forgotten who. Shortly thereafter, she became a licensed facilitator for my Get Clients Now!™ program. I was impressed with her business savvy and coaching ability, and in 2003, I tapped her to join the faculty of Get Clients Now! University. In 2005, I selected her to become the first ever Director of Licensing and Training for my company, a position she held for four years. At the same time, Joan maintained an active coaching practice of her own, as well as leading numerous workshops, and developing workbooks on work/life management and delegation.

During the time Joan worked with me, she co-authored her earlier book, *Women, Work, and Autoimmune Disease: Keep Working, Girlfriend!* I was thrilled with her perspective that work, rather than being just another burden to carry while dealing with a chronic illness, could actually be a bright light in one's life. Continuing or returning to work can provide you with personal fulfillment, needed income, an important role to play, and a welcome distraction from your health worries. But you need guidance and support to follow this challenging path.

I know just what it feels like to try to function as a competent professional when you don't even feel well enough to put on your shoes. I remember once being on my way to a speaking engagement, feeling so miserable that I had a complete meltdown on the sidewalk, and had to stop and call one of my coach friends for a pep talk just so I could pull up my socks enough to continue on.

This book can serve as that "coach friend" for you. In its pages, you'll find inspiration, wisdom, techniques, and camaraderie—everything you need to carry on, survive, and rebuild during and after a health crisis.

As I write this Foreword, I am myself recovering from an accident. My broken right hand is in a splint, and I'm taking pain medication for my injured shoulder and jaw. I've been working reduced hours recently, due to the discomfort of working with injuries, time out for physical therapy exercises, and traveling to multiple medical appointments. I've been vividly reminded of the need for this book.

This time around, during yet another health crisis, I'm in luck. I have Joan's wise words to help me work, recover, and thrive despite my injuries. With this book in your library, you can have that guidance too.

C.J. Hayden, MCC, CPCC
Business coach and author of *Get Clients Now!*
and *50 Ways Coaches Can Change the World*
San Francisco, CA

Acknowledgments

This book may have been written by one person but it was supported by a small village. I am enormously grateful to Noreen Henson at Demos Health for her belief in the potential for a second book, and her willingness to work with me until I got the topic right. Marketing manager, Tom Hastings, and managing editor, Dana Bigelow, have been patient, responsive and encouraging during the book launch phase. They made a somewhat stressful time less far less stressful.

Practically speaking, the manuscript would not have been in the shape it was in when I turned it over to the publisher if not for the diligence of Lenore Costello. Her keen eye for grammar, and her feedback in places where I had questions, were invaluable. I thoroughly enjoyed the partnership that evolved as we worked our way through the book.

Business from Bed was not born in a vacuum, but in a series of conversations after *Salmonella* poisoning reminded me of the very worst flare-ups when I was ill with Crohn's Disease. For their friendship, ideas and interest, I thank Clara Griffin and Tish Kashani. You were there with me during pivotal points proving, once again, that two—or more—are better than one.

This book would not have been nearly as rich in content if not for the clients and interviewees who gave their time and allowed me to ask questions about an aspect of life that few feel comfortable discussing. You move and inspire me, and for your input and genius I am forever grateful. Thank you for putting your trust in me.

I am thankful for the friends who listened when fear and doubt plagued me—and they did. Sue Rasmussen and Susan Bock were always available on the other end of the phone when I got hit with a doubt-monster. Carly Anderson gave me much needed friend-relief (as well as the space to "not talk" when I was buried in the book) and my husband simply said, "I know it will be great." Sheila Dixon, founder of Women in Business Investing in Success (WBIS) in Northern Virginia, made sure that I started referring to myself as an author, encouraging me to be proud of my work. Karen Vandermaas Walsh not only guided me through the discussion about disclosing at work, she has been a cheerleader, too, introducing me to people in her network who could lend a hand or make a business connection. Many others cheered me on whenever I posted a book milestone on Facebook. Your "likes" and comments buoyed me up more than you may know.

My mentors are many. Some know they are mentors and some speak to me through their books. I am especially grateful for the guidance, friendship, and partnership of C.J. Hayden over the past 10-plus years, and for her coaching last year, the year of "figuring it out." We were both surprised when my answer to the question, "how will I scale up?" turned out to be through the writing of this book.

I remain grateful to the health practitioners who helped me on my healing journey. They include Janet Golden, Greg Cherney, Julia Marie, and Dr. Craig Ennis. You helped me find my way without being heavy-handed.

Finally, even in their quietude, my family grounds me. My son, Matthew Ury, lights up my life. I always enjoy hearing how your mind works and what you have to say. My husband, John Linzy, is simply and always "there," and stepped in at the eleventh hour to help me review the proofs. Thank you for keeping us afloat while I dived into this book. My parents gave me the foundation on which to build a reasonable life, and I have to give a shout out to my brother, Eric, who is always good for a few laughs.

If I have missed anyone, please forgive me.

Prologue

FROM HEALTHY TO SICK AND BACK AGAIN— MY THIRTEEN-YEAR COMEBACK STORY

One day, or over a series of days, weeks, or months, you realize that something is wrong, really wrong. You go to the doctor, or hospital, and have a bazillion tests taken. You begin to use up sick days and one day the doctor says, "You have X. And X is not something we know how to cure. However, we do have medicines you can take, or machines we can hook you up to that will have their own side effects. But it doesn't matter; we have nothing to actually make this thing go away."

If you've been healthy all your life, this is not good news! It's so not good news that you're likely to fight it. If you're like me and you believe that the circumstances in your life are within your power to change, then by God, you will conquer this. If you are less willful than I was, once diagnosed you'll say, "Okay, give me the meds." Either way, your first response is, "Make me feel better!" No matter who you are, or your approach to life, the traditional response to a sudden loss is denial and abject fear. And, no matter which side of the spectrum you're on ("Screw this, I can make this go away" or "Okay, tell me what to do so I can feel better"), your journey has only just begun.

The road ahead involves many personal and important decisions. You've just gotten a swift kick in the pants accompanied by a command order: It's time to pay closer attention to what you are doing and where you are headed. If you heed the call of your body, you and your life will never be the same, and you won't just be impacted physically. Your mind and spirit and the definition of who you are as a human being are now up for close examination—and that's the good news. Will you kick and scream and make everyone else miserable (including yourself), or will you rise to the occasion and make the most of a challenging situation? Truthfully, you will probably do both. That's okay. That's to be expected. Hopefully, you will discover how amazing you are, and your life is.

7/15/92—Journal Entry

Probably my last day in the hospital… I am present to sadness, not at leaving the hospital, but for my body and the pain it went through, for my 1st major illness, for a condition that will [require] care to prevent recurrence, and for myself who must return [to my life] and transform some ways that haven't worked. How will I do that? What choices will I make, what ways of operating will I have to give up, what will I have to alter? What can I keep? What will I have to discard?

Shortly after I was given the diagnosis—initially Ulcerative Colitis and later, Crohn's Disease—I learned that the cause is unknown, it's considered a chronic disease, and that there is no cure. This was a problem for me, as I believed that my will and intention could change anything I put my mind to. I believed that my circumstances were malleable and that I was the driver in my life, no questions asked. Stubborn, stoic, determined, and frightened: all adjectives you could use to describe my response. At first, these qualities were problematic. I resisted the diagnosis with everything I had.

Crohn's Disease impacts your intestinal system in ways that are absolutely un-ladylike. In the midst of a flare up that could last anywhere from a couple of weeks to a few months, the location of the nearest bathroom was always at top of mind, night sweats often required a complete change of clothing, and food became the feared enemy. Yet, the drive to work, to engage with people, to do something that makes a difference, never subsided.

I was in the hospital twice in 1992, the first time in July and the second time in October. Instead of slowing down at work after that first hospital stay, I returned to my job in my dual role as store manager and regional training manager for a national bookstore chain. I'm sure I must have regained some strength and shown some improvement, since the doctor authorized my return to work. I am also sure that I used up most of my sick time, so I would have been motivated to return to work. That summer I was asked to add the role of Acting District Manager to my list of responsibilities and I said yes. It was an exciting opportunity, one I'd never imagined getting, and I did not yet know just how sick I was to become. Neither did my manager. Now I had three distinct roles in the company: as Manager of my own store, as the Western Region Training Manager, and as Acting District Manager for Southern California.

As Acting District Manager, I was required to periodically visit different stores throughout Southern California. On one such occasion, I was so symptomatic that I had to run to the bathroom every 15 minutes or so. I was mortified. I remember leaning on the steering wheel of the company van as I drove 60 miles to yet another store, but I kept going. I didn't stop. I didn't say no, I just kept going. I couldn't believe that by applying the power of my will and my mind I couldn't overcome this. I didn't realize that caring for my body would have to become my top priority, and that doing so was critical. By the time October rolled around, I was a complete wreck. My body was weak, I had dropped ten pounds I couldn't afford to lose and I was in a great deal of pain.

The summer and fall of 1992 marked the beginning of a long journey back to health, vacillating between stretches of remission and times of extreme discomfort and pain. When a new District Manager was finally hired in January of the following year, I was not only released from my responsibilities as Acting District Manager, I was soon relieved of the Training Manager position, too. I lost a lot of ground when I was ill, and it took all of my energy to get through the busy holiday season. Between my illness and my extra responsibilities, I was not able to keep up with the duties associated with maintaining and running my store. In January, shortly after the new District Manager was hired, the company merged two divisions and only one Training Manager was required in my region. I imagine it was a relatively easy decision for management to make. I was left with my job as Store Manager, and nothing else. I was devastated.

Things were changing in the company, and it became clear that I'd not regain access to new opportunities anytime soon. I left seven months after my demotion to take a management position with a new company, where I thought my chances for regaining the same level or responsibility were greater. It did not pan out: I hated the company and had no interest in staying. It was time for me to leave retail and look for a different kind of career path.

For the next six years, until I started my coaching business, I struggled to find a new career direction, moving through four more jobs. Two of the job changes were precipitated by another round of disability leave. Once the most acute symptoms started to subside, and I could think of something else besides the pain, I asked myself "What do I need to change in my life? What am I not paying attention to?" One time my internal guidance said it was time to walk away from an unhappy marriage. More often, my guidance nudged me to look for another position, hoping to get closer to the level of fulfillment I felt when I was training new bookstore managers.

In 1995 I was "let go" from one of those jobs the day after returning from a 10-day disability leave. I was 39 years old. In the wake of the shock I was highly motivated to ask, "OK, what do I *really* want to do with the rest of my life? What are my options?" A wonderful book called *Do What You Are*, by Paul D. Tieger and Barbara Barron-Tieger, started me on the path towards coaching, but not for another few years and three more jobs.

FROM EMPLOYEE TO SELF-EMPLOYED

At first, I set my sights on becoming a career coach who would focus on helping people navigate career transitions. I was good at that! In 1999, when employed at a very nice pay-the-bills job, frustrated by my lack of progress towards my career aspiration, I hired a career coach and committed to one year of coaching and to the dream of launching my coaching business. I finally launched in September 2000, just three months after my last—and longest—disability leave. I had recently remarried and had just relocated to another county in Southern California.

I started my business slowly, buoying my start-up efforts with a part-time, 6-month temporary assignment as a benefits manager. I landed my first paying client in December 2000. By the time I finished the temporary assignment, I had five coaching clients. I was happily on my way.

Even though I have never had to take another disability leave since starting my business, there were times when my symptoms would flare up. Sometimes they would be mild and other times more severe, requiring that I work under the covers from the comfort of my bed, literally. Fortunately, I worked with most of my clients by telephone, so I could take care of my body when needed. With a lap desk, a portable phone with a head set and a computer, much is possible. (My husband reminded me that my needs prompted him to install Wi-Fi in our house at that time, as this was before "everybody" had it.)

Even when my energy was low, and my brain was feeling foggy from the symptoms or the drugs I took to help manage my symptoms, I still managed to be present with and for my clients. Coaching them actually gave me a reprieve from the pain as my attention was turned away from me and towards them. This always astounded me, and I most certainly appreciated it. However, during the most severe flare-ups, I had no leftover energy to do anything creative. My marketing efforts and business development tanked during these times. My heart and mind often wanted to do more but my body could not. It was a frustrating time in my business. Nonetheless, I never questioned the choice. The path of self-employment was much more attractive than full-time employment, for the following reasons:

- I have complete control over my physical environment.
- I can set my coaching schedule around my personal needs: health, family, doctor's appointments
- I can potentially earn more per hour—by far—in the time I have available for work

- I am able to do work that matters, that is meaningful to me and those I work with
- My boss—that's me—is understanding and adjusts her expectations as needed. She is less concerned about the time I put into work than she is to the quality of my work, my earning capacity, and my sense of satisfaction.

FAST FORWARD—2012

Now 20 years since the onset of my illness, I am happy to report that the major symptoms associated with my illness have been in remission for over seven years, since early 2005. When people ask me what I did that eventually put my symptoms into remission, I venture a guess that the same stubbornness that initially created a dangerous situation in 1992 may have had something to do with it, that and my never-ending quest to course-correct when life required it. Even though I eventually accepted the potentially chronic nature of my illness, and became a "compliant" patient regarding my medical treatment, I never was able to buy into the idea that my body didn't have the capacity to heal itself. In truth, I don't know, with certainty, why or how my symptoms went into remission. What I can say, for sure, is that I feel quite strong now. My body still does little things here and there—whose doesn't?—but my ability to modulate my energy is second nature now. I don't think about it. I just respond and adjust.

I write *Business from Bed* from my home office. I don't have to work from bed anymore and I don't very often. However, I can regulate the temperature of the room I work in. I can wear comfortable clothing. I can move around from desk to sofa to kitchen table, as needed. I don't attend early morning networking meetings unless they are highly interesting and compelling. But I can.

I started my business as a career coach in order to assist mid-level professionals in successfully navigating transitions from jobs that were not satisfactory to others that would feed their souls. It wasn't long before I started working with people in mid-level positions who wanted to navigate their way out of a job and into a business. Shortly after I started my business, I was introduced to two programs, initially through books by the same names, first *Work Less, Make More®*, developed by the late Jennifer White, and then *Get Clients Now!*™ by C.J. Hayden. Both offered templates for business success that I found compelling and sound. (You'll read more about these programs and their creators at different points in the book.) As my business—and I—evolved, I noticed that my clients changed. I stopped coaching people in career transition and started coaching business owners.

My own "comeback plan" took thirteen years. The road back to health was a rocky one, indeed. Between the uncertainties associated with my illness, and the meandering road to discover my real passion, I've fallen and come back more times than I can count. Though I would never presume to know what your life's course should or will be, it is my wish that the *6-Step Comeback Plan* will ease the way and shorten your trip.

All my best,

Introduction

*It's actually the inability to have access to the community that
makes people with disabilities less happy...*
—SAMUEL BAGENSTOS, LAW PROFESSOR AT WASHINGTON
UNIVERSITY IN ST. LOUIS[1]

Illness, typically considered a sign of weakness, is a taboo subject in the business environment. Business owners keep their conditions hidden so that their customers keep their attention where it should be anyway, on the value and quality of the business service or products. Employees throughout the ranks keep their health issues hidden, fearing loss of employment. *Yet, illness is a part of life, not just for a select few, but for millions of people around the world. Business from Bed is,* among other things, a book meant to normalize an aspect of life that many determined professional men and women endure in isolation and silence.

In our society, discussions around sex and money are fraught with hushed whispers and false bravado. Illness is equally problematic as a topic of discussion—several business owners who were asked to share their experiences for this book declined, even though anonymity was assured if requested. Luckily, many others were willing to come forward and share their "comeback" story with me, so that I could pass their wisdom along to you.

Bob, a successful rainmaker in the real estate business, was one of those people. I met him at a networking meeting just a couple of months after he re-engaged with business, following treatment for Non-Hodgkin's Lymphoma. I asked Bob how his illness and subsequent treatments impacted his business. Here is what he said:

> Chemotherapy was absolutely exhausting. I was unprepared for the physical effects, not the nausea but incredible fatigue, bordering

on anemia. At times I couldn't get out of the chair…It took a good 6 months after chemotherapy ended to drain all the chemicals from my blood. There were times when I felt I was ready to hit the ground running and start again and I couldn't. I would completely run out of steam. Even though they told me it would take that long to get back to normal, I kept expecting it would be faster.

YOU ARE NOT ALONE

Nearly 1 in 2 Americans are living with some kind of chronic illness[2] (133 million in 2004), and 60%[3] (approximately 80 million) of those are between the career-building years of 18 and 60. In 2006, the Census Bureau reported that the U.S. had more than 20.7 million "non-employer businesses,"[4] otherwise known as self-employed business owners. It stands to reason that a significant portion of entrepreneurs and would-be entrepreneurs will have to deal with the challenge of facing a health crisis and managing their business at some point in their lives. If you're like most people, you probably rarely talk about your problems, and may end up feeling isolated—like you're the only one dealing with this issue. However, these statistics indicate that on any given day, there are many more people like you, who are also working from "under the covers" in the comfort of home or bed, because it's the only way they can earn any kind of living while attending to their health.

NEDI'S STORY

After spending almost six years close to home and in bed with severe pain associated with persistent endometriosis, Nedi, a talented musician and a single mom of two teenage boys, finally regained enough strength to get out of bed and back into life. Unbeknownst to me at the time, her first step at getting back in the game was attendance at the first Work Less, Make More® workshop I ever led. She was thrilled to have enough strength to get out of the house and think about her career again. However, she feared that she'd have to settle for another life-killing job instead of pursuing her passion as a songwriter and musician. Fortunately, the message of the workshop emphasized the positive aspects of pursuing your dreams by focusing on your unique gifts.

Encouraged, Nedi tapped into her musical talents and started by teaching piano to the children in her neighborhood. Slowly but surely, she regained her health and began to take on more students. She went from feeling helpless and dependent to becoming self-sufficient and capable. Not only that, she reclaimed her first passion and is, as of this writing, doing "live" concerts via Facebook from her home studio, something that would not have been possible when she and I first met. Technology advances have made the most unlikely dreams possible for people who must remain vigilant about safeguarding their health.

Nedi's experience reflects that of countless creative, entrepreneurial men and women who must stay close to home, often in bed, for an extended period of time as a result of a painful, energy-draining illness. She told me that if she could change one thing about her experience it would have been to tell the truth about her situation much earlier, and to have asked for help. It is Nedi and people like her that inspired me to write *Business from Bed*.

WEAK NO MORE

In our modern culture, there is neither tolerance nor time for illness. Our business lives have been designed so that we must be continuously engaged, lest we feel like we're falling behind. We set aggressive agendas that even the healthiest people have difficulty managing. Most days are filled with more to do than time to do it, and reliance on our ability to continuously produce dominates. I'll wager to guess that cave people had more down time than we do, and they had far fewer resources at hand! But I digress.

It's time that those of us who must slow down for our health stop seeing ourselves as weak and ineffective. As a matter of fact, the opposite is true. Such determination is a sign of commitment to two seemingly conflicting priorities: career success and managing one's health. If necessity is the mother of invention, finding a way to work, even if from bed, is most certainly an innovative solution for those who need to do so.

TECHNOLOGY INCREASES OPPORTUNITY

When Rosalind Joffe and I wrote *Women, Work, and Autoimmune Disease*[5] in 2007, technology offered many alternatives to traditional employment, but the flexibility we had then was not as prolific as it is today. In just five years, the advancements in "tele-technology" have increased significantly. Business owners, and many employees, can more easily work from anywhere in the world under a variety of circumstances. Why shouldn't working from bed be one of those circumstances? Timothy Ferris, author of the wildly popular *The 4 Hour Workweek*, opened up doors for office employees to enjoy a flexible lifestyle, too. It is time we bring the same opportunity to the countless men and women who, at some time in their lives, need the same level of flexibility in order to manage their health.

ILLNESS IS A VEHICLE FOR TRANSFORMATION (THE RULES HAVE CHANGED)

Most of the people you'll meet in the book saw their health crises as opportunities to reflect on their lives, as well as their businesses or careers. During the recovery period, the "truths,"—guiding values that previously dictated behavior—often came under close scrutiny when ill health made it impossible to continue operating at the normal warp speed.

No matter what your symptoms are or how they have impacted you, you are in a unique position to discover previously hidden strengths and to course-correct for a more satisfying, authentic future. If you are like me and the people I have coached and interviewed, you have already started reviewing different aspects of your life: your relationship with yourself and with your loved ones, your assessment of priorities, the way you approach opportunities and challenges, and everything you believe about business and success. Debbie, a physics scientist who you will meet a few times in this book, explained it like this. "I realize I have to change my entire approach to life and the world from what it was 'before' and, especially, to what it has been like since being on disability. Somehow I've come to believe that everything 'should' be a struggle and that life is about tense periods of being out in the world interspersed with retreat away from it. I definitely need to 'chill out.'"

RECOVERY AND INTEGRATION

Many of the people I talked to reported that when they moved away from the most acute period of pain and ill health back towards wellness, a connection with their inner wisdom often diminished. I experienced this, too. Alongside the excitement—and relief—that naturally accompanies the restoration of health a new kind of tension arises. Impatient to get back to work, your mind starts to reassert its control. Warning: your mind is not always the most reliable authority on what is ultimately good for you. It is the control center for survival. It is good with facts, information, and memory but it is also oriented towards fear. It houses self-recriminating messages. It is often a source of pressure rather than a source of comfort. Too much reliance on your mind, and you are likely to find yourself disconnected from your heart, your body, and your soul, back to old habits of behavior and thought.

Peggy, a mortgage loan officer and former coaching client, spoke to me a few months after she finished three rounds of chemotherapy following a double mastectomy. She described the inner war between body and mind, as follows:

> I tried really hard; I tried to convince my mind and my body that I had to do this. I didn't have any money coming in at all. It was hard to get out of bed in the morning. It was hard to be positive. It was hard to keep track of things… I kept trying to convince myself I was capable, but you know, I wasn't.

> There were times I'd turn on my computer, but I just had to go to bed. Body trumps. You can try, but body will win…. The biggest frustration has been getting my body and mind to coordinate with each other. My mind thinks my body can do more than it knows

it can. I think I have more energy than I do. I plan things and I make my to-do list and my body says, "Are you out of your mind?" That's the thing, my energy is slow to come back and I try to push it. Your body won't let you push it; your body will only allow you so much.

When you are ready to rebuild your business—and your life—it may not be the same as before you became ill. You are not the same. As you move away from illness and towards wellness, you straddle three personas:

- The way you used to do things, and who you were before the health crisis
- The person you are now, perhaps more vulnerable, somewhat weakened, yet strong and resolute
- The person you will become as you integrate your insights and physical recovery with new growth

The key to rebuilding your business life while also maintaining a connection to improved health and well-being is to find a way for your mind and your body to live in harmony. If you have been feeling ashamed and lost, *Business from Bed* will restore your sense of self-worth and self-confidence, traits that are often diminished when you feel like you have lost control of your body.

WHO THIS BOOK IS FOR

Business from Bed is primarily directed towards men and women who have moved through the most acute phase of their illness and are ready to make their way back to their business on a more "normal" schedule. In addition, it has the potential to help employees at all levels of a company. Some readers may even be motivated by their illness to abandon the previous career path entirely, and start anew. The stages of recovery across all three groups are common; the specific questions that you ask as you redirect your life and business/career may be different. Where useful, I have offered specific guidance and questions for each of the three groups.

The people you will meet through this book have been where you are now. Some have fully recovered from their health crisis. Others are still dealing with severe or intermittent symptoms. They are strong individuals, determined to find a way to make a reasonable income doing meaningful work, and to remain faithful to the lessons learned. Their various illnesses or injuries lasted anywhere from six months to six years or more. The full recovery period, especially the recovery of their previous level of business success, often took longer. They have endured and survived a wide range of health issues, including cancer treatments, physical injury, heart disease, and multiple sclerosis, to name a few.

Some of the people I interviewed were comfortable sharing their stories with their names attached. Others wished to remain anonymous. In those instances, I've used only their first names or changed their names entirely. In all cases, they were generous with their time and open about their experiences.

WHAT THIS BOOK ADDRESSES

Business from Bed is a crossover book. Other books on similar topics focus on either the restoration of health and well-being after a health crisis or specific illness, *or* on matters pertaining to business success. *Business from Bed* addresses both. It shows you how to answer the questions that those who have walked the same path struggled to answer for themselves.

- How can you put your business/career back together in new ways that are more satisfying and sustainable?
- What are your options for earning a living if you have to stay close to home or in bed?
- If your health crisis has prompted you to change your business approach, how do you figure out what to do?
- How do you deal with sudden vulnerability when you're used to being independent and capable?
- What do you tell people about your illness, when do you tell them, and who do you tell?

- How can you plan and set goals when you're not sure how you will feel the next day?
- How can you rebuild and maintain your business—or reignite your career—while also remaining mindful of your health and well-being?
- How do you deal with the emotional impact of having expectations of yourself that you cannot fulfill?

In addition to the life experiences shared with me by my clients and the business owners and employees I interviewed, *Business from Bed* includes practical guidance. Most of this guidance is delivered in question form, giving you greater access to your own intelligence and wisdom. As you will learn, if you haven't already, your health setback has the potential to steer you towards decisions and actions that you'd not previously entertained. Some people become more practical and strategic; others become more innovative and bold. Most people do a little of both. Regardless, if you have been making decisions according to someone else's standards of success, I say it's time to live by your own.

THE 6 STEPS OF THE COMEBACK PLAN

The 6 steps of the comeback plan are designed to help you successfully integrate your emotional and physical healing with the practical aspects of rebuilding your business or career. Specifically, Steps 1, 2, and 5 will show you how to deepen and maintain your connection to the "new you." These three steps will help you tame the impatience that is likely to arise as you experience the ebb and flow of physical, mental, and emotional recovery. Steps 3, 4, and 6 will assist you in taking the practical and tactical steps needed to rebuild your business or career, one that is better aligned with your updated values and sensibilities.

Step 1: Beyond Survival, Rising from the Ashes

Step 1 meets you in the most vulnerable place of all—between life as you knew it before, and life as it is now. In order to move ahead, you need to address the fears associated with your illness. You will need to understand the nature of the journey and what threatens your comeback. In this step you'll be invited to disconnect your self-identity from your illness and to separate fear from fact. You'll meet people who got stuck, and people who used their illness to shift their points of view about themselves and others, enabling them to return to business with more personal integrity.

Step 2: Embrace the New Normal

Having disconnected your self-identity from your illness, you can look ahead more freely towards rebuilding your business and your life. Step 2 is all about the "ideal life." You'll be invited to open yourself up to reconstructing a business/career that incorporates your values, includes your dream of the "perfect day" and "perfect work," and enables you to tap into your greatest gifts and talents. As you'll see, manifestation of the ideal may take a few years to come to fruition. However, if you don't imagine your ideal in detail, it's less likely to materialize.

Step 3: Back to Business Under "New Management"

In Step 3, you will turn your attention from inwardly focused questions toward "real world" concerns: How will you rebuild your business or career without undermining your health, and where should you begin? Starting with six foundational business questions, you'll integrate the new insights gained in Step 2 to devise new solutions.

Step 4: Ask for Help

Ah, yes, the Achilles' heel of every self-sufficient person: the sudden need to ask for help. Every person I interviewed mentioned just how difficult their new dependence was, at least initially. They also admitted that it was one of the gifts of their health crisis. Learning to ask for help changed their relationships—and their ability to recover—in positive ways. Nonetheless, it's not as simple as just asking. There are important questions to answer: who can help, how can they help, how can you respond to unsolicited help, what about privacy or potential threats to the business (or your career) when word gets out, etc. These questions and issues are addressed in Step 4 so that you can decide who does what and when.

Step 5: Slow Down, Don't Move Too Fast

When you are recovering and rebuilding, one of the biggest frustrations and greatest opportunities lies in the struggle between your mind and your body. Step 5 will help balance your drive to get back to work with your wish to live a healthier life. You will learn why it is a better long-term strategy to return to work at a slower pace than you may like, and the role that adrenaline plays in the war between mind and body. You'll be introduced to "body breaks," which are specific techniques you can use to modulate your energy throughout the day. Finally, you'll also gain insight into how to answer one of the more difficult questions of any health crisis, "How do you know when to yield to your body and when to push through?"

Step 6: Build Capacity, Organize for Success

Step 6 builds upon Step 5. Once you have established harmony between mind (goals) and body (needs), Step 6 will show you how to develop a "Master Planning Schedule" that will help you maintain this harmony. You will learn how to plan and set goals when health and energy waver, without veering from your priorities.

HOW TO READ THIS BOOK

You may be tempted to skip steps or start in the middle. However, unless you're absolutely certain that you are fully on track with rebuilding your business/career without any residual fears associated with your illness, I encourage you to start at the beginning with Step 1. Having coached entrepreneurs and other career-minded people for over a decade, I know how tempting it is to skip the internal work and get to the more tactical work as quickly as possible. However, I can assure you, it does no good to develop a marketing strategy for your business if you have not built the emotional foundation to support it.

Robert Kiyosaki, most famous for his book, *Rich Dad, Poor Dad*, wrote another book which I like just as much, *Before You Quit Your Job*. In it, he tells the story of how and why his first business failed. It was not because he could not sell his product. It was because he had failed to put the structural foundation in place that would support the sales. As a result, the business grew too fast and his business crashed. *Your body is your structural foundation and your number one business asset*. Building a business, when it is not yet strong enough to support your efforts, will only bring the same disappointment Kiyosaki experienced.

I've included a variety of questions and exercises in each chapter. Since this is *your* comeback story, I encourage you to answer the questions and do the exercises that seem most worthwhile. You might skip some only to come back to them later. If you recognize questions you've answered before, you may want to answer them again. Experience and time will change some responses and reinforce others. It's worth finding out which ones persist regardless of changing circumstances, and which have changed.

I suggest buying a notebook, journal, or other record-keeping tool, as there will be many prompts throughout the book to jot down your ideas and make important decisions. You can use a note-taking or record-keeping software program, if you prefer.

Even though the 6 steps are presented in a linear fashion, don't be surprised if the answers and solutions you seek pop up at unexpected moments. Give yourself the gift of curiosity and trust in "right timing." Enjoy the journey!

Step 1:
Beyond Survival, Rising from the Ashes

There is no intelligence in torment.
—GUY FINLEY, *THE SECRET OF LETTING GO*

As often happens when a major life event changes you, a line has been drawn in the sand. There is life as you knew it before, and life as it is now. You have been unwittingly thrown into the hero's journey, a journey you would not wish on anyone, yet one that has the potential to change your life in positive ways. It is likely to be one of the most challenging journeys of your lifetime, one that requires you to garner strength you never knew you had, while pulling you into the deep shadows of the greatest fears you have ever known. Will you survive or better yet, will you—and can you—thrive? Yes, you will and yes, you can. In order to do so, it helps to understand the nature of the journey and what threatens your revival.

Susan Bock, one of the entrepreneurs interviewed for this book, explained it like this: "I'm so grateful for what happened because if it had not my life would be very different today, and I'm not sure it would have been better....If I have the courage to ask new and different questions, and I'm willing to uncover what's in there, that means I hold the key. But, I have to have the courage to unlock the door and let the light in."

YOU ARE NOT YOUR ILLNESS

While an acute health setback will certainly affect your life, it does not have to define your life. I read an article in which a young man who had been severely impacted by a difficult illness said of his situation something like this: "I can focus my attention on the 5% of my body that is not functioning well, or remember that 95% of my body is just fine." His proclamation stopped me in my tracks. He was right. When pain or illness exceeds what you can easily tolerate, it sucks up all of your attention, so much so that you lose sight of what does not feel like pain. When Eckhart Tolle, author of several popular books devoted to personal and spiritual transformation, was counseling a woman living with Lupus on a show with Oprah Winfrey, he said something similar, "There is well-being in your body even when other areas are in pain—put your attention there."[1]

I am ambivalent about this. I think that part of the healing process does include acknowledging the pain. It is incredibly difficult to deny your pain when it feels like it has taken over every cell in your body. However, it is also true that whatever you put your attention on expands. In the interview, Tolle suggested the following to help this woman disconnect her *identity* from her illness.

- Stop talking about it with friends and family.
- Only talk about it with your doctor, or with people who can help you change your situation.

Tolle's recommendations are extreme as a singular strategy. However, I do think that if it has become habitual to talk to about your illness in just about every conversation, it would be healthy to interrupt yourself and talk about something else, instead. I'll say more about this later in the chapter.

THE ASSUMPTIVE WORLD SHATTERS

All plans are built on assumptions, consciously or not. People marry assuming that their love will last a lifetime. They accept jobs assuming that they'll be able to remain employed as long as *they* want. Entrepreneurs start businesses assuming (or at least hoping) that they have the ability to exert enough influence and control to achieve a reasonable portion of the goals they set. The list goes on. Even when you do plan for contingencies you can't possibly plan for all of them. To try to do so would make you crazy and impede progress.

Whatever we set our sights on and wherever we go, our bodies transport us. They are our vehicles, and we rely on them. Unless one has been sick since childhood, most people perceive their bodies as allies, and silent ones at that. We also take them for granted. Consequently, when they "misbehave" and interrupt our plans, it is as disruptive as any major force of nature. When this silent partner of yours suddenly develops a voice and demands your attention, plans and dreams must be altered to account for it. We don't like that.

We become attached to our plans, especially those that promise to deliver rewards we strongly desire. Ten days before the manuscript for this book was due to the publisher, we lost power in the midst of a sudden, unexpected, twenty-minute rain storm. I had established a schedule and a timeline for those last ten days, and was looking forward to the coming week. Without any thought that it would be otherwise, I assumed that I would have access to electricity and the Internet, never imagining another

3

scenario. For the three days the power was out in my area, I was a mess. My dream of sliding into home base, happy and blissfully finishing this book, was threatened.

I tried to be calm as my husband and I figured out where we could "plug in" (he works from home, too), and how we'd keep ourselves cool and fed as the temperature rose to 100 degrees in the afternoon. But I wasn't. As much as I tried to take it easy, I could not. In addition to the mental energy being exerted to put together the "contingency plan," I was attached to my picture of how it was going to be. I hung on for dear life to the normal routine, to anything and everything that resembled the picture I had invested in. I was determined not to alter the plans that had been set around this particular deadline, including the vacation set for the day after the manuscript's due date. Nor would I allow myself to take a single day off to relax. I got caught in a comparison trap, between the plans I had made and the reality of the moment. I've been disappointed before so I know that I would have eventually adjusted if required to. But, boy, was it hard in the moment!

A LIFE INTERRUPTED

Charlene, a composite of several women I've met over the years, portrays a scenario that is somewhat extreme but not uncommon. Hers is a story of a life interrupted by illness and compounded by a divorce. When she became so ill that she couldn't care for herself and her two children—and needed to leave an unhealthy marriage— she moved into her mother's home. Many of the business owners I interviewed did not reach a point when they had to move back home, yet the fear lurks in the background. Illness increases the threat of poverty, emotionally and physically. The knowledge that you may have to depend on others threatens to chip away at your sense of security, if not consciously, then unconsciously.

"Charlene" has two degrees, one in Business Administration and the other in Fine Arts. She suffers from Fibromyalgia, which makes her joints ache and her often tired and depressed. Except for disability benefits, she has no other income. She enjoyed a different lifestyle before her divorce. Her ex-husband was a good provider, so when her second child was born she gave up her consulting business and became a stay-at-home mom. Before she became ill, Charlene had a good life: good friends, a nice car, two children, and an emotionally distant husband, (almost) everything she ever wanted.

No matter how sick she was, Charlene never thought she would get to a point of not being able to support and care for herself. She misses her old life and feels very isolated. She doesn't leave the house much, except to run errands and take her children to their various activities. She paints, is creative, and has a good mind for business. She connects with old friends on Facebook, enjoys working on her computer, and sometimes takes online classes to learn something new. She has ideas about ways she can work from home (she'd love to start a new business), but she has been unable to figure out what makes sense due to her physical limitations.

Charlene's circumstances are difficult, if not dire. She wants to change her situation and feels she has the ingredients to do so. She also fears that she can't. Her illness, her pain, the divorce, coupled with the move back into her mother's home and her reliance on disability benefits, have shattered her belief in herself. Her physical limitations are real. Her financial situation is real. But, they are not insurmountable. She is smart, she has useful skills, and she is able to take classes, paint, and work on her computer.

BEWARE OF THE COMPARISON TRAP

One of the greatest threats to your recovery is the degree to which you compare life today with life as it used to be, especially when life before you became ill seems insurmountably better than life since. The way Charlene views what happened may be more threatening to moving forward than her circumstances. She is stuck in the fairy tale. She views her life before she became ill as a better life. Yet, in the midst of her story we notice the presence of a husband who is emotionally distant. Standing on the outside, looking in, we may sense a home environment that was less than healthy and ideal. We don't know why Charlene got divorced; we only know that she did. Making the decision to close her business to become a stay-at-home mom was not inherently unhealthy or unwise, but it did create a potential for financial vulnerability she did not anticipate.

We know that Charlene knows how to set goals and take action—she has two degrees—and that she is creative and extremely capable. For many years, she thought of herself as someone who could tackle anything that came her way. The severity of her illness and its impact on her ability to support herself has taken its toll. She has fallen into a hole of the darkest circumstances she could ever have imagined for herself.

Every time Charlene compares her circumstances today with those of her past and comes up short (I used to be a such-and-such and now I am so-and-so), she reinforces her doubt in her ability to change her situation today. She maintains the belief that what she had before was better, and what she has today is worse. She does not realize that by holding onto this belief, she reduces her ability to make positive changes.

Without changing her circumstances, Charlene *can* change the tone of her story.

- Instead of romanticizing the past, she can paint a more balanced picture of her marriage.

- If she became ill during the marriage, and her illness contributed to her eventual divorce, she could see it as the best thing that could have happened.
- She can most certainly draw real strength from her past accomplishments and innate gifts and talents.
- Even if she can't leave the house with any degree of frequency, she has the energy to pursue that which interests her: taking classes, doing things on her computer, and creative activities.

Charlene is stuck in a "comparison trap." Like the young athlete who can no longer play after a severe injury, the greatest obstacle to healing and moving on is his or her insistence that the life of the athlete is the only possible avenue for fulfillment. Others, like Magic (Earvin) Johnson, former star player with the Los Angeles Lakers basketball team who was diagnosed with AIDS in 1991, use the break with the dream to redirect their energy and talents in a new way. If Charlene were to put her attention on what is okay in her life, it would help lift her energy. She may not know what to do yet, but optimism will make it easier for her to explore her options.

I do not mean to say that you should not lick your wounds, feel sorry for yourself, roar with frustration, and otherwise mourn the life you were enjoying. As a matter of fact, the healing journey is well served by your retreat into a period of grief. In her book, *Tough Transitions*, Dr. Elizabeth Harper Neeld identified these type of initial reactions as essential to any significant life transition (which the healing journey most certainly is), the stage she calls "responding."[2]

Table 1.1 lists common responses to a severe health set back. Which ones have you experienced?

If you go back and re-read Charlene's story you will see many of these responses in her story, including betrayal, victim, breakdown,

TABLE 1.1
Typical Responses to a Health Crisis

Typical Emotional Responses	Fear
	Betrayal
	Broken Hearted
	Victim
	Regret
	Impatience
	Rebellion
Typical Physical Responses	Breakdown
	Weakness
	Sleeplessness
	Exhaustion
	Pain
	Foggy Brain
Typical Social Responses	Embarrassment
	Shame
	Guilt
	Indignation
	Pretending
	Withdrawal
	Isolation

pain, withdrawal, and isolation. Even though they are normal responses, Charlene is stuck; she hasn't progressed. She knows it, too. In order to write her own comeback story, Charlene has to find a way to let go and move on. It is time for Charlene to release the past, to tell the story one last time, and then use the positive elements in her story to help design her future.

DISMANTLING THE COMPARISON TRAP—OBSERVATION

Now it is your turn. As uncomfortable as it is to face the thoughts that keep you stuck, I want you to walk your "pity trail" one more time. This time, you'll do it with purpose. Rather than judging and comparing the present to the past without discernment, you are going to first, observe, and second, release.

Dismantling the Comparison Trap— Observation

When you compare your life today with your life before your health setback, what do you say to yourself and to others? Use the following questions to fill in the details:

1. What were *you* like before you became ill?
2. How were things better?
3. What were you able to do without much effort?
4. What do you miss the most?
5. How much money were you making? How much are you making now?
6. How many hours a day were you able to work?
7. What were your relationships like? (Consider family, friends, colleagues.)
8. How would you describe your lifestyle before you became ill? How would you describe it now?
9. What other comparisons have you been making that I've not covered in the questions above? Write about those.

After you answer the questions above, do something that feels really good. Take a walk, call a good friend, watch one of your favorite TV shows, enjoy a tasty snack, drink a full glass of water, or take a nap. When you're ready, come back and continue on.

DISMANTLING THE COMPARISON TRAP—RELEASE

Review your answers to the questions above. For each of your responses, I want you to consider that you may be romanticizing or idealizing the past. Remember, this is a normal response, especially when what you are facing in the present feels overwhelming and difficult.

1. Was there a down side to the comparison situations you described?
2. Was there a cost to the "better" life that you have overlooked or omitted?
3. Were you omitting or minimizing some aspect of the story of your life before illness that would offer a more complete or accurate view of the past?

Once you have a more complete picture of the past, it will be easier to minimize the influence of an ideal that has hindered the healing process. Bob, the real estate agent you met in the Introduction, has a different view of life now than before his year-long ordeal with cancer treatments.

I'm optimistic and confident I can get back to an acceptable level of productivity, but not by doing it the same way or with the same mindset as in the past. I think some of the motivations that drove me to the business were not healthy motivations—things I had to prove to myself—things that made whatever success I did achieve come with a high price. I was always pushing and aware of what I ought to be doing, feeling guilty about what I wasn't doing.

Previously, I would make other people wrong, which is not healthy. I can be judgmental and very stubborn. There are many practices in real estate that are just plain stupid. Quite honestly, they don't serve the public, yet [agents] engage in them over and over due to custom and habit. A prime example is the open house. Clients want us to do them, but it's only good for the realtors. No one buys from an open house. I couldn't convince [sellers] that the open house was a waste of their time, and then I'd get frustrated. I see now that my own inability to explain my thinking to them was the problem, not them. That's just one example. So, when I talk about rebuilding the business, but in a different way, it's not going to come at the expense of my own health.

Trying to [understand] the relationship between those attributes and my illness (non-Hodgkins lymphoma) led me back to asking why I have a need to be right, to wonder what happened in my childhood that made me feel that way. If you stay with it and try to make it better, you start to ask yourself certain kinds of questions that can make your life better. So I look at [my illness] as a positive experience.

TIME FOR A EULOGY

Symbolic rituals are useful means for letting go and making more room for a different future, a created future rather than a given future. Once you have busted the mythology in your comparison story, garnered its gifts and uncovered its truths, you may want to perform a eulogy. Your eulogy can take many forms. Review the four approaches below and choose the one that is most interesting to you. If you want to do more than one, then do!

Draw a Picture or Create a Collage

Draw a picture or create a collage from magazines, using words and pictures that express the thoughts, feelings, and facts of life before and after illness. Using two separate pages or one single, larger sheet of paper divided into two sections, create a picture of the "before" life and your "current" life. Include all details in your comparison story, romanticized and realistic, to create your picture. When you are done, put them aside for a day or two, but no more than that. Take them out and look at them again. Gaze at your images with meditative eyes. What do you notice? Is there some detail or image that is newly revealed you'd not noticed before? Are there any similarities between them?

Review Your Story One More Time

Read through your answers to the questions in "Dismantling the Comparison Trap—Observation" again. It is your story. Don't try to change anything. Just be with it. If they come to you, ask more questions and listen for the answers. Make additional notes if you feel called to do so. When you're done with the review, put your notes away. You can file them, or shred them and recycle the paper. If you decide to shred your notes or otherwise discard them, imagine they are leaving you alone, in peace, calm, comfort, and ready to move forward.

Tell Your Story to Someone You Trust

When someone bears witness to your story, it can be quite powerful for a couple of reasons. First, when you talk out loud you hear things differently than when the story cycles in your head unfiltered. Second, when you tell your story to someone else its hold on you often dissipates. What has been stuck in your head, swirling around you like a bottomless whirlpool, is released, much like what happens when you open a jar for the first time.

In order to make this method successful, it's important that you choose your witness carefully. Select someone who will listen with all their attention, and without judgment or interruption, who has the capacity to see it as a story, and not "the horrible truth." Tell your witness that you are not seeking their feedback, or even their sympathy, and that you only want them to listen. Ask them to hold your story in strict confidence. If there are some potentially horrific elements in your story, prepare your witness for this fact. Finally, tell your witness that it is your intention to release your comparison story in order to make room for the creation of a different future. Ask them to listen with the same intention for you.

Dissolve the Energetic Epicenter

Read your answers to the questions in "Dismantling the Comparison Trap—Observation" out loud into a recording device. Then play it back. Close your eyes and listen from a comfortable position, either in a comfortable chair or lying down on a sofa or bed. To prepare yourself, you may want to take a few deep, relaxing breaths first, in order to increase your receptiveness.

As you listen to your story, pay attention to your body. See if you can detect the "energetic epicenter" for your comparison story. You'll know you've hit upon it when you feel some kind of tightness in the area. Is it in your shoulders, in the middle of your back, around your solar plexus (just below your heart), in your gut, in your forehead, or elsewhere?

Once you sense your attention is finely tuned to the energetic epicenter, hold your attention there as long as you continue to detect some energy. If needed, stay with it even after the recording of your comparison story has stopped playing. Observe it: What color is it, how big is it? How dense does it feel? Has it moved to another location? Is it growing bigger or growing smaller? Has it disappeared?

If your attention moves away from the energy center at times, it's okay. Just bring it back. When you notice that the energy mass associated with your comparison story seems to have disappeared (or as much as it's going to for now), prepare to open your eyes. Take a couple of deep breaths and when you are ready, open your eyes. You might want to get up and shake your body or walk around for a bit.

Regardless of which method you choose to release your comparison story, when you are done you are likely to feel somewhat drained, yet lighter and more optimistic about your future. If you notice any residual emotions, it does not signify that it didn't work. As with any cleansing process, it is wise to allow your body to rest and recover. Drink a full glass of water, take a nap, go outside and go for a short walk, or sit somewhere comfortable. A full night of sleep will do the trick, but don't push it. If it takes a couple of days before you notice renewed energy and optimism don't fight it, trust it.

RIDING THE EMOTIONAL PENDULUM

Human beings experience a range of emotions. We have good days and we have bad days. We all know what it is like to be around a person who, on any and all days, talks primarily about the tragedy of his or her life. We also know the person who, no matter how difficult things are, wears a rosy smile, amplified by a cheer in their voice that somehow rings false, insisting that everything is fine. The range is not problematic. Getting stuck on one side or another is. Figure 1.1 shows the extreme edges of emotional response, and how they are commonly expressed.

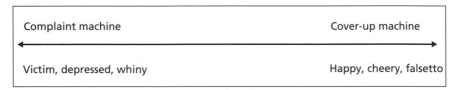

FIGURE 1.1
The Spectrum of Human Emotion

Denying the full range of emotions is more threatening to your recovery than responsibly expressing them. At my last job, when I was feeling particularly grouchy, it was much worse if I withdrew into that grouchiness than when I found a way to express how I was feeling without taking it out on the people around me. It was easier to release my grouchy disposition when I could admit how I was feeling to a co-worker. I knew that the grouchiness was leaving my body when I started to feel the heat of the emotion in my face and a little sweat under my armpits. Telling it like it was in that moment—not with an intention to escalate or hang on to it for the rest of the day, but with an intention to simply share it with another—enabled the "grouch" energy to move up and out of my body, thus returning me to an improved sense of well-being.

There are many ways to release negative emotions. Another person might have stepped out of the office and called a spouse or good friend to let off steam. Someone else might head out for a walk around the block. Yet another person might take a break, get into their car, close the windows and yell it out. Your approach to managing the emotional roller coaster is personal. You must find out what works best for you.

CHANGING "IT IS TRUE" INTO "IT USED TO BE TRUE"

When you say that something is true in present time, you inadvertently perpetuate the unwanted circumstance. You strengthen its hold on you, mentally and emotionally. It doesn't matter if something was true yesterday. If you no longer want it in your life, you can change "I am" into "I was" or "I used to be." You can change "I never" into "In the past I did not...." You can turn "they don't" into "they didn't."

Bob made this kind of switch once he realized that the way he thought about his clients, blaming them for his inability to communicate effectively with them (a form of "they don't"), was not true. Essentially, he turned "they never listen," which is present-tense, blame-oriented speaking, into "I wasn't able to explain my thinking to them." He took responsibility and stopped perpetuating the myth. Instead of "I have no money," someone like Charlene could say, "I have less money than I used to." The first statement would keep her stuck in a victim's role. The second statement is merely a fact, with no blame, guilt, or resentment attached. Can you feel the difference between the two statements?

Talking about unwanted circumstances in the past tense can be tricky if you are still experiencing symptoms associated with your illness, or an unpleasant memory is fresh. You would be right to wonder how you can talk about it in the past tense if it is part of your life today. The truth is, you can't. But you can become mindful about how you may be limiting your healing through the use of "it is" language.

If you are in the habit of repeating negative statements about you and your life to yourself and out loud to others, regarding them as facts rather than judgments, you have mistakenly equated yourself with your illness. You have decided that it is you and you are it. Below you'll find a short list of common (misguided) judgments you may recognize. On the right side I offer alternative statements that are more empowering, without sugar-coating the situation.

TABLE 1.2
Modifying the Self/Illness Paradigm

Common Judgments	Alternative Statements
I am a failure.	I have had a health set back.
I can't because I'm ill.	I don't want to, thank you OR I would like to, and I wonder how I can.
I am not worthy.	I may not be able to do as much as I have in the past but my life still matters.
I am weak.	It takes incredible strength to get up each day. I am strong.
I am not fun to be around anymore.	I can laugh and cry with the best of them.

When you change your perspective you clear a new pathway for growth, growth that is built on an internal sense of strength, love, and appreciation for yourself and what is possible in the future. Whenever you feel stuck or unhappy about your circumstances, return to Step 1 in the comeback plan. Select the exercise that you think would help you disconnect your sense of your self-worth and well-being from your illness.

5 Things to Remember, Try, and Discard

5 Things to Remember

1. You are not your illness
2. You are not alone
3. You have done nothing wrong
4. You can emerge from this
5. Your body is your ally

5 Things to Try

1. Patience
2. Appreciation
3. Change "I am" to "I used to"
4. Speak your truth without apology or blame
5. One new habit or practice of your choosing

5 Things to Discard

1. Heroic behavior
2. Negative self-talk
3. Restrictive assumptions
4. Quest for perfection
5. The comparison trap

Step 2:
Embrace the New Normal

I still am who I am, and a Genie in a different bottle
is still a Genie.

—NEDI, SINGER AND SONGWRITER

Truer words were never spoken. They point to an essential "law of life" for your comeback story. You are unshakably "you." Regardless of your circumstances, your values, your unique attributes, and your gifts and talents are relatively consistent. They may be buried, they may be misguided or misused, but they exist. In fact, discovering, embracing, and expressing your uniqueness can take a lifetime. A health setback provides you an excellent opportunity to review, revisit, and shed crusty old layers of misaligned choices.

When I speak of misaligned choices, I do not mean that you are to be blamed for behaviors and choices you have made so far. You have always made the best choices possible in any given moment with the insight and information at hand. Yet, you cannot escape the impact of education, cultural traditions, parental feedback, and peer pressure on life-level decisions. Why not use this recovery period to review and reflect upon your needs and aspirations?

Nedi realized that no matter what else she does in life she is, at heart, a singer, and songwriter. Through her illness, she discovered that no matter how many times she made choices that masked or buried her true essence, her well-being and sense of joy would only be possible through the pursuit of a career that allowed her to express her gifts. The same sense of purpose and determination that guided her can guide you through illness and back towards a well-lived life.

The avenues through which you express your uniqueness can take more than one form, yet some are more fulfilling than others. We see evidence of this in the stories of uncountable men and women who started working in one field and, through some unpredictable happenstance, become more effective and fulfilled in another field entirely. Successful lawyers, such as John Grisham and David Baldacci, discovered the writing muse within and became best-selling authors of courtroom dramas and mystery novels. They are not alone. Many people engage in more than one fulfilling career in their lifetimes.

Jack, an actor, turned to the field of coaching and used the same set of skills he used in acting to help people play a bigger, more rewarding life-game. Jack loves play, he loves words, and he loves to provoke. That actor-turned-coach is using the same set of skills that made him a moderately successful actor (a genie in a different bottle is still a genie), but in a way that is ultimately more satisfying and has the potential for greater success. Jack, the actor, still gets to play to an audience. Jack, the coach, gets to tap more directly into his true desire—to move audiences to play a bigger game.

Laurie Erdman, a successful vice president of sales administration for a large company, was diagnosed with multiple sclerosis (MS) mid-career. She eventually turned her self-directed health and wellness recovery program into a business to help others with MS minimize their symptoms through diet and lifestyle changes. Here's what she had to say about her jumping off moment.

> At the time I was diagnosed with multiple sclerosis, I was the vice president of sales administration for a public company. It was a big and stressful job. In many ways [my condition] did not impact my ability to do anything—it wasn't that I couldn't type, or see the screen, or anything like that—but for me it was a wake-up call.
>
> I was diagnosed two days before Christmas. It was December 2009, the year we had the big snow storms. Between the snow storms and vacation, I was out of the office for three weeks. I came back and I remember walking down the hall and wondering, "What am I doing here!?" It wasn't in the sense of "What am I doing in this office building?" but "What am I doing in the world?" It felt like an out of the blue question. In truth, I'd been asking it for quite a few years.

I asked Laurie, "Was it the convergence of these significant events at once that gave rise to the question? Would you have had that thought anyway? Or, do you think that question 'dropped in' with the additional factor of the diagnosis?"

> It was a question I asked myself a lot. "What is my purpose here, because I don't feel like this is it?" I was one of those people with serial employers, and even though I was with this company for 8 years, I had many different positions. I was always looking for something that was the right fit, which was the right thing for me. So, I was always asking that question but it had a much deeper, more profound weight to it when I asked it that day... because of the realization that I could not continue working so hard at something that wasn't satisfying. It was like my body had been whispering for a long time, and now it was screaming, "You can't do this anymore!" So, the weight of the question, "What am I doing here?" felt very different than it ever had before. It was the wakeup call to actively do something different, but it didn't give me the answer of what at the time...A big part of the gift was the freedom it gave me to leave the corporate world.

As you'll see when you read Step 3, Laurie has taken the same set of skills and talents that made her successful in earlier jobs, and combined them with a deeper sense of purpose and passion, and mixed in additional education and training to create a business that allows her to have complete authority over her work, her lifestyle, and her health.

For sake of this discussion, the genie is your "essential self." The bottle is the way you choose to express your gifts, either through your business or your job. If you realize that you can no longer do what you were doing before you became ill, or that you can—and want to—but will need to approach things differently than before, then you are in a most exciting place. To help you in this journey, I offer you a treasure hunt, a return to your essential self.

WHAT MAKES YOU HAPPY?

People who are thoroughly engaged in activity which hits the right mix of difficulty and novelty and feedback are the happiest.
—MIHALY CSIKSZENTMIHALYI, *FLOW*

What makes you happy? Why would I ask you that? How can I talk about happiness when pain and confusion persist and your livelihood is on the line? I talk about it because happiness and health are inextricably linked. When you feel relaxed and happy, your breaths are deeper and richer in oxygen content, bringing more oxygen to your cells, and increasing your potential for healing. When you feel unhappy, your body naturally contracts, reducing the flow of oxygen to your cells and your organs.

In recent years, happiness has become an increasingly popular topic of discussion, perhaps because people are feeling less control over their daily circumstances. According to Sarah Pressman,[1] an assistant professor of psychology at the University of Kansas and a Gallup senior research associate, positive emotions are unmistakably linked to better health, even when taking into account a lack of basic needs. The inverse holds true as well: Negative emotions [are] a reliable predictor of worse health. Her findings are based on data from the Gallup World Poll with adults in more than 140 countries providing a representative sample of 95 percent of the world's population. The sample included more than 150,000 adults. Participants reported emotions such as happiness, enjoyment, worry, and sadness. They described their physical health problems—such as pain and fatigue—and answered questions about whether their most basic needs like food, shelter, and personal safety were adequately met.

Martin Seligman, who has been a leading voice in the research regarding the factors that influence happiness, and the impact of happiness on health and well-being, discovered that many of the aspects of life normally correlated with happiness are, in fact, basically irrelevant. Factors such as climate, education, money—even health—have been shown to have little or no effect on happiness. What, then, positively impacts our sense of happiness? Seligman points to three areas of life where we have "voluntary control"[2]:

1. Degree of satisfaction about the past (gratitude and forgiveness)
2. Optimism about the future
3. Happiness about the present (including status of flow, meaning, and purpose)

I covered the first influencing factor in "dismantling the comparison trap" in Step 1. In Step 2, I'll present several avenues of discovery through which to access the third factor, after which the second factor, optimism about the future, should rise on its own.

Joelle's return-to-work experience illustrates the impact of one simple change towards a more centered, happy life.

When I returned to my job as an administrative manager after a two-month disability leave, I noticed something remarkable. After being out for two months I had slowed down. Even though I was really happy to get back to work and join my peers once again, when we went to lunch I was astounded by the difference between my posture and theirs. A small group of women headed out the door at 11:45 AM, bodies pitched forward, moving as fast as they could to get to their cars, to get to the restaurant, to get seated on time, to order as quickly as possible with hope that the food would arrive giving them plenty of time to eat it, only to return to the office at the same pace, with bodies pitched, once again, in the forward position and feet moving as quickly as possible.

I was no longer like them. Something had changed in me. With my head and shoulders comfortably seated on top of my torso, I was inclined to move at a much more relaxed pace. Noticing I was falling behind, I did pick up the pace so that I could keep up. Even so, my head remained centered over my body and I vowed never to move at that pace again. I felt certain that by slowing down and moving with a more centered posture, it was better for my health and well-being. I was not special. I was like them. However, while I was out on disability leave, my life came to a complete stop. I had interrupted what had been a steady dose of hurry-up just to enjoy my lunch break. I could see and feel the difference.

Imagine the compounding value of making many small adjustments to your actions, thoughts, and behaviors. I dare say you owe it to yourself. It is your right—and it is your obligation—to do what you can to live a life that gives expression to your talents and gifts, that aligns with your values and maximizes your health. Laurie Erdman refers to such practices as "radical self-care." She likens them to the instructions adults receive at the beginning of every air flight: put the oxygen mask on yourself first; you'll be much more helpful to others. When I imagine a world in which people are doing work they enjoy, with people they like and in an environment and manner that supports health and well-being, I imagine a world where stress is minimized, the soul of the individual is nourished, and the well-being of families, communities, and even countries, are enhanced.

CHANGE STARTS WITH YOU

Will you be a leader in your life, or will you continue to sublimate your desires, values, and dreams to obligations, survival, and fear? Do you have, or will you develop, the capacity to take a strong stand for your life, even if doing so is not popular? By popular, I do not mean well-liked. I mean commonplace, ordinary, homogenized, and "normal." The greatest role models and leaders of our time have developed this capacity: Mother Theresa, Oprah Winfrey, John F. Kennedy, and Lady Gaga are just a few. We all have an opportunity to be leaders of our own lives. Why not you?

It is not easy. Transformation never is. Steeped in survival instincts, there is great fear associated with standing apart from the crowd (our tribe). The crowd does not have to be large. It can be the person sitting across the table from you, or the voice of an authority figure in your head. To be true to you requires a good dose of healthy leadership capacity.

TOOLS FOR SELF-RECOVERY

If you equate success with the achievement of tangible, measurable results, you may have difficulty with the slower pace of the inward journey. Yet, having been ill myself, I suspect you can see just how infrequently you stopped to smell the proverbial rose when you were working at a faster pace. When you are poised to get back to work and rebuild, it will serve you well to continue to nurture your inner life so that when you are back to "normal" you will remember that there is much more to you than business and work.

In order to stay connected to the richness of life as you reemerge and recover, it helps to gather tools that will tap into your creativity. The "tools" of childhood are especially helpful. I am referring to particularly silly tools, like crayons and construction paper, to more grown up tools, like journals and colored pens, and everything in between. If it has been years since you sat on a floor with paper and crayons at your feet, give it a try now. Can you feel the six-year-old within sitting in your adult body? (If it hurts to sit on the floor, by all means, sit at a table—or in bed!.) There is nothing more healing—and fun—than using the tools and skills of a first grader when you are reinventing your life.

During my second hospital stay in 1992 I surprised myself. Although I considered myself to be absolutely lacking in artistic expression, I had the wherewithal to ask my then-husband to bring several artistic tools to the hospital when it became clear I was going to be there for a while. I asked him to bring a previously unused journal, a set of colored pencils, a pen, and my tarot cards. (Not having a strong connection to any religion, the cards served as my means for tapping into what others would call a connection with something greater than me.) Every day I, the "un-artist," found myself drawing pictures in my journal and illustrating the selection of Tarot cards for the day.

I was only in the hospital for 10 days, but my fear level was often high. Plus, 10 days in a hospital room, with limited access to the outside world (laptops and cell phones were not yet as omnipresent as they are today), and hours when neither family nor friends were present, gave me a lot of time to dwell in my own fear thoughts. The journal, the Tarot cards, and my amateurish drawings helped me stay centered and focused on my intentions—to avoid a blood transfusion, gain weight, and get well enough that I could eat regular food again and go home. An added bonus: My son, who was seven at the time, joined me in the doodling process. Three of my drawings are shown in Figure 2.1. This is what artistic looks like in my world!

If you haven't already, I encourage you to buy a journal or a notebook to document your journey. You can use it to catalogue your thoughts and experiences, and do the exercises in this book. The following are tools you can choose from to add color and dimension to your work:

- Crayons and colored pencils
- Plain and colored paper

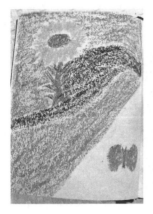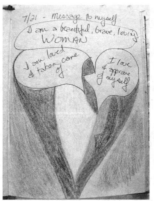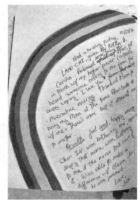

FIGURE 2.1
Joan's sketches and doodles while in the hospital, 1992

- Magazines
- Photographs (yours or someone else's)
- Note paper
- Blank journal, 3-ring binder or artist's notebook

YOUR IDEAL LIFE

"If you can dream it, you can achieve it."
—WALT DISNEY

When I worked for Brentano's books in Century City, Los Angeles—before I became ill—I envied the people standing in line at the ticket window of the movie theater just outside our doors on my way to my 45-minute lunch break. I thought about how marvelous it would be to get to a place in life when I could do that, too. Of course, I had no idea if these people were between jobs, worked at night, or were between acting gigs. All I knew is that I wanted that in my life.

Eleven years later, a year after launching my coaching business, that wish became a reality. I was working with C.J. Hayden's

28-day marketing plan template outlined in her book, *Get Clients Now!* In this system you are allowed one "dessert" action.[3] (Hayden describes the dessert action as something you do that will make you more effective in everything you do, in marketing and the rest of your life.) When it came time to select my "dessert" action, I remembered my wish so I committed to taking one afternoon off a week, during the workweek. On most of those afternoons I went to see a movie. I was excited. Not only did I reach my 28-day business goal, which was to gain two new coaching clients, I was able to enjoy a lifestyle of my own design. As unattainable as that dream may have seemed when I was working for Brentano's, through the twists and turns of my life, the freedom I sought to work on my own terms materialized.

Walt was right: If you can dream it, you can achieve it. I would add that it helps to believe that "it" is possible. I wouldn't draw a straight line between the two events in my life, but I do give credence to the power of a desire. Let's find out what your perfect day, perfect work, and perfect lifestyle would look like.

The Perfect Day

I get up when my body is ready, usually around 7:00 AM, or when the sunlight starts to filter into the room. I don't normally schedule my first client call until 11:00 AM. When I was ill with a Crohn's flare up I could not do anything reliably before 9:00 or 9:30 AM. As gross as it is to admit, during a Crohn's flare up I had to go to the bathroom, and urgently, several times in the morning. I did not dare attempt to do anything before my body "emptied out." This is what made working at a job so difficult for me. After I started my business I could set my hours accordingly. Later, after my symptoms went into full remission, I discovered that keeping these kinds of hours suited me very well. As an introvert and a writer, allocating the morning to business projects that are either creative or task-oriented works very well for me.

Looking back to the days when I was a store manager, I see now that the hints regarding my ideal day were already in play before I became ill. I loved getting into the store at 8:30 AM, 90 minutes before we opened. It allowed me to focus in solitude for a full hour before the rest of the staff showed up to prepare to open at 10:00 AM. Conversely, I disliked the days when I worked the afternoon/evening shift, requiring that I walk into the store at 1:00 PM, smack into the middle of a busy store.

What Does Your Perfect Day Look Like?

Use the questions below to develop your vision for your perfect day. *Do not describe what life is like now, but how you would like it to be in the future.* The questions are divided into sections to help you think about this from a couple of angles. They are further divided to distinguish between what your main concerns will most likely be if you are a business owner or an employee. You may find some of the questions easier to answer than others. Don't be alarmed if you don't know how to answer all of the questions right now. Later in the book, in Steps 3, 4, 5, and 6, we'll delve more deeply into some of these questions, and you'll be able to revisit them again. For now, answer them as best you can and keep your answers on hand when you work in other chapters. Remember to use the creative tools you've selected to develop a full-blown, colorful, multidimensional picture of what this day would look like.

- Ideally, when would you wake up?
- How would you like to spend the first one to two hours of your day?
- At what time do you want to start working?
- By when do you want to stop working?
- How much time do you spend on your own; how much in the company of others?
- What's your favorite part of the day? Why?
- What feels more like play than work?

- How are you spending your evening hours?
- How are you spending your free time?
- How many days a week do you work?

The perfect work—for business owners

- What skills or talents to you get to use every day?
- How would you like to answer the question, "What do you do?"
- Is anyone helping you run the business? If yes, what are their roles? Do they work alongside you or in another location?
- What product or service do you sell?
- Who, or what cause, are you impacting?
- What do you never have to do again?
- How much revenue is the business generating?

The perfect work—for employees, managers, and executives

- How would you describe your ideal job?
- What skills or talents do you get to use every day?
- What is your role in the company?
- What is the company culture like?
- What is the nature of the business you work for? Service, manufacturing, mission, for-profit, non-profit, etc.?

The perfect work—for everyone

- On average, how much money are you bringing home each month? Each year?
- How do you spend your discretionary money; i.e., money not used for necessities?
- How much money are you able to put aside for future interests or needs such as travel, education, retirement, etc.?

The perfect work arrangement

- Where do you work? From home, at an office, or a little of both?
- What are the people like where you work?

- Do you work in an open environment with people all around you, at your favorite coffee shop, or in a quiet office where distractions are few?
- How do you reach your income goals? Is it completely up to you? Do you earn a steady paycheck? Do you have a reliable income base, plus the ability to earn commissions or bonuses?

Summarize Your Findings

In answering these questions, you've unearthed a great deal of information that will help you develop your vision for your ideal life. To summarize, make note of the following before moving on to the next section:

1. Were any of your answers especially surprising to you? If so, what stood out most?
2. Between 0 and 100, with 0 being not at all, to what degree would you say you are already living and working according to your ideal day in your ideal business or company?
3. What would you like to explore further?

ROLE MODELS

As you get older it is harder to have heroes, but it is sort of necessary.

—Ernest Hemingway

Another good way to catch a glimpse of your ideal life is to think about the people who inspire you, because of what they do and/ or how they live their lives. You may know some of these people personally, you may have only read about them or seen them on TV—or YouTube—and they may be alive now or have passed on long before you were born. Regardless of their status, you can tap into these role models as you rebuild your business, career, and life.

Furthermore, if they possess qualities you desire, then they possess qualities already in you. Just as you cannot see flaws in another that you do not possess yourself, you cannot see brilliance in others that you don't possess, either. Start by answering these two questions:

- Who inspires you now?
- Who inspired you when you were young?

When you select your role models, include at least one person who is in your life now, at least one who is alive even if you have no direct connection to them now, and two to three other people—living or dead—personally known to you or not, real or not.

When I was a young girl, two of my role models were fictional characters in two of my favorite books. One was "Caddie Woodlawn" by Carol Ryrie Brink and the other was Karana, the young narrator in the "Island of the Blue Dolphins" by Scott O'Dell. I read and re-read those books several times between the ages of 9 and 12. In college I took a course in children's literature, and treated myself to both books one more time. I found I was still inspired by their stories.

Discover Yourself through People You Admire

After you have identified four or five role models, answer the following questions for each of them.
- Why have you selected him or her?
- What about this person most inspires or inspired you?
- What qualities or behaviors does this person exemplify that you'd like more of in your own life?
- What qualities or behaviors does this person exemplify that you have seen glimpses of in yourself?

Review your responses for each of the role models you selected. Do you notice any themes or overlapping qualities in your selected role models? If so, what are those themes or qualities?

Research the Life of Your Role Models

Now it is time to dig a little deeper. Imagine you are interviewing these four or five people. What would you most like to ask them in order to better understand their life stories? Your questions may be identical or different for each person. After you have developed your interview questions, it's time to do some research. If your role model is alive and known to you, contact him or her and ask if you can meet with them. Tell them that you'd like to ask them a few questions. By all means, tell them they have been a role model for you. They might be embarrassed but they'll also be flattered.

If your role model is alive but not someone you know personally, look for sources of information about his or her life on the Internet, on TV, or in books. Whichever means of research you choose, keep your interview questions close by and see if you can answer them through your research. If your role model is in the public eye consider looking for an opportunity to attend an event where he or she will be speaking, or a program he or she will be attending. You may not be able to do this right away, but even if the event is several months or even a year from now, it will be worth it. Can you feel the excitement of anticipation, just thinking about it? If your role models are fictional characters, like a couple of mine were, you can craft your questions and then look for your answers in the story (books and movie characters qualify).

As you conduct your interviews and do your research, document your findings in your working journal, in a document, or on a poster board. If you find pictures, quotes or articles by or about your role models, cut them out, and make them part of your collection.

If you have forgotten what you were like and what interested you as a child, doing these exercises and answering these questions can help you remember. They are stored in your body and in your memory. This is one way to recover and reclaim it.

As you are filling in the profiles of your role models, think about the following:

- How are they just like you?
- How are they different from you?
- If they are different, do you think they are different because they possess different values or goals than yours (which is quite okay) or because they have developed a skill that you haven't yet developed?

Add your observations to your profiles.

VALUES MATTER NOW MORE THAN EVER

By now you have likely uncovered some long-forgotten dreams and unveiled desires for the life you want to create. I hope that you are falling just a little more in love with yourself, too. To round out the picture of you, it's time to clarify and own your unshakable values. Your values act like a well-tuned barometer. When you are aligned with them through action, you will find yourself naturally drawn towards opportunities, people, and activities that are well-suited to you. Similarly, you will be naturally repelled by opportunities, people, and activities that don't match up. When I have asked business owners to articulate their top values, they universally report that by understanding what motivates and drives them, it is much easier to make decisions about their business and their lives:

- It becomes easier to know who belongs on their team and who does not
- It is easier to choose marketing activities and approaches that are authentic, as well as effective
- It is easier to direct the growth of their business

■ It becomes easier to set boundaries around their time and with people

■ It is easier to understand why some situations put them at ease and others make them uncomfortable.

People who have experienced a health setback report that one of the greatest gifts of their illness is their recovery of values that they had forgotten, the importance of which they never fully understood. Here's what Peggy, a customer-centered mortgage broker, said about the importance of embracing her values when she returned to work shortly after her last chemotherapy treatment.

Question: What is different about your business now?

I needed to be around people with a positive attitude. I decided I need to make sure I'm working with the values that I hold. I started a new program where I get up in the morning and ask:

1. *Who am I?*
2. *What are my core values?*
3. *What am I doing to live up to them?*

I guess I discovered that life does end, and is too short. I might as well make the best of what I've got. I want to offer a positive attitude to the people around me. I want to feel good. If I go against my core values I don't feel good. In my industry it's very easy to go against core values, thinking it's not a big deal. We'll just say, "It's done all the time," but I can't do it. I have to stay true to my beliefs.

Question: How are you different now?

I've always wanted to help everybody. Wanting everybody to like me and wanting to be able to do everything for everybody really hindered me in some respects. I know now that it's a disservice when you give people false hope. This is one way I'm being more honest with myself. Now, when I'm uncertain about a client's situation, I ask others to look at a deal with me. Fortunately, I now work in a company where people are happy to look at deals without trying to steal the business. (It wasn't that way in the last company I worked for.) Once I look at a deal, and have others look at the deal, and I realize that there is absolutely no way I can help someone, I go back to the client right away and let them know the situation. I discovered that it may not be what they want to hear, but they prefer to hear it upfront rather than down the line.

Values Help Reduce Anxiety

When working with Debbie, who was suffering from the painful, isolating effects of chronic pancreatitis, and felt anxious about her social skills at school (she is taking classes to launch a second career as a high school physics teacher), I suggested that she look to her values for guidance. I hoped that by getting in touch with her values that her anxiety would be reduced and she'd feel more at ease with herself, whether she was being social or not. She chose six words to represent her values: grace, prayer, acceptance, curiosity, appreciation, and honesty.

Before we met again, she went through her magazines in search of images that represented those words. In addition to pictures, she found simple quotes that embodied those five words for her, one quote for each word. When we next met, she confessed that she almost didn't do the exercise. Her negative self-judgments about her artistic and creative abilities almost stopped her. Fortunately, she persisted and did the exercise anyway. I thought the results were beautiful. In the end, Debbie thought so, too. (See Figure 2.2 for her collage depicting the word "curiosity.")

By doing the exercise, something she already knew about herself reemerged. Debbie feels most peaceful, happy and "at home" in nature. She lives just a few blocks from the beach but rarely gave herself permission to walk down to it, to drink in the beauty of the shore.

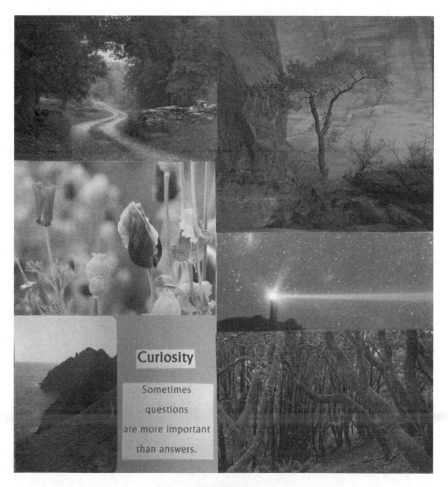

FIGURE 2.2
Debbie's Collage—Curiosity: Sometimes questions are more important than answers

What Are Your Values?

When you compromise your values you risk compromising your health and well-being. Sure, you can get away with it for a while, but doing so will slow down healing. Those I interviewed concurred; their health crises were wake-up calls. Sometimes your values whisper to you in a moment of quiet contemplation. At other times, they hit you over the head if you're not paying attention. No doubt you have recalled or uncovered some of your values already. Now is the time to capture them. Following is a two-step process through which to uncover or clarify your top five values.

Step 1: Using the life categories below (feel free to substitute words that represent them better), make a list of 3 to 5 specific values or practices for each life area. It will be best if you develop your lists on separate pages. Your pages can be any length you want. Your lists can be linear, or you can use mind-maps or your favorite software program. If any of the proposed life categories hold no meaning for you, eliminate them. They are only suggestions.

Universal Life Categories

- Work or Career
- Health
- Family
- Social
- Spirituality or Religion
- Recreation
- Hobbies
- Financial Welfare or Security
- Lifestyle
- Education

Step 2: Now go back and review your lists. Lay your lists out side-by-side. Using a highlighter or a colored pen or pencil, make note of the words that stand out for you in each of the life categories. Pay particular attention to the words that appear on more than one list.

Table 2.1 shows examples of values or practices that one could list for two of the life categories, Work/Career and Health.

TABLE 2.1
Example of Step 1—Values and Practices for Business/Career and Health

Business/Career	• Respect for everyone • Recognition of my contribution • Environmentally friendly workplace practices • Reasonable working hours—no more than 45 a week
Health	• No more than one sugary snack a day • Eat three meals a day • Go outside at least once a day, even if only for 5 minutes • Pay attention to my gut reaction before accepting invitations. If my "gut" says "no," politely decline

Upon review of the value and activity lists in "Values and Practices for Business/Career and Health," we can extract the following values from the Business/Career and Health categories, as shown in Table 2.2. Note that the four activities listed in Table 2.1 on the "Health" list would be considered practices, not values. However, when we look more closely, we can see that these activities could reflect the values listed in Table 2.2. Remember, the values and words used to describe them are personal selections. You might come up with different words to describe the values for the same practices.

TABLE 2.2
Example of Step 2—Values and Practices for Business/Career and Health

Business/Career	• Respect • Recognition • Environmentally-friendly • Reasonableness
Health	• Practice • Moderation • Discipline • Discernment

Step 3: On a new page, write down—or type up—the value words that have shown up in more than one life category. If you don't feel as strongly about some of those words you can leave them off your values list.

Step 4: Review your culled list of value words and prioritize them. Select the 5 values that resonate most strongly with you. You'll know the difference. If you're not sure, just pay attention to your body. Does your energy increase when you look at a word, or decrease? When it increases, it points to what is more important or positive. When it decreases, it points to something less important or distasteful.

Some people need to hear themselves speak in order to tune in, with accuracy, to their inner guidance. If this is you, find someone to share your values list with. Don't ask for their input. Ask them to listen so you can hear yourself speak. The only input you might ask is whether or not they noticed a change in your voice or energy. Remember, these are your values, and yours only.

Mapping Your Top Five Values onto the Wheel of Life

A "Wheel of Life" diagram is often used by coaches and other helping professionals as a tool on which clients can visually illustrate their relative satisfaction with the different life areas. You can use the same tool to create a visual map of your values as they are reflected in your chosen life categories.

First, draw a circle and divide it into 10 equal slices (or fewer if you are mapping fewer life categories) and label each slice with a life category name. Then, using a scale of 1 through 10, where 1 indicates you have veered far off-course from your values in that category and 10 means that you are expressing your values in every way you can imagine, you would draw a line at that approximate location. The closer to the middle of the circle your line is for that life area, the greater the gap between your top 5 values and your expression of those values in that area of life. See Figure 2.3 for an illustration of what a "Wheel of Life," minus the life categories, would look like.

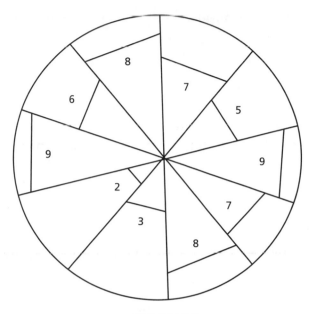

FIGURE 2.3
Sample Wheel of Life

If, after you map your values onto the "Wheel of Life," you notice feeling badly about those areas you scored less than 5 or 6, remember this: at first the truth may discourage you, but in the end it has the potential to transform your life. If you were not aware before, you are now. With awareness comes the possibility of change.

Put Your Top Five Values to Work

You don't have to tackle all "problem" areas at once. To start making changes, select one or two life areas where you'd most like to narrow the gap between where you are now and where you'd like to be. How do you prioritize? Do you start with the life area to which you've assigned the lowest number or do you select a life area where the gap isn't as great, but you feel positively motivated—and capable—of starting an associated practice now? Most people would instinctively choose to tackle the value with the lowest numbers first, but I invite you to decide using a different lens: what would be easiest for you to do, *and* have the greatest positive impact?

I'll explain. When you take steps to positively increase the alignment of your actions and in one life area, you are likely to improve alignment in other areas, too. Why? There are no walls within you. What you do for yourself in one area has the potential to elevate your life in other areas. So, you don't have to work as hard as you would think to raise your scores in all life areas. You only have to identify two or three life areas for which you will launch one new practice each to benefit the entirety of your life.

For example, let's say one of your values is "financial security," and you equate peace of mind with financial security. What if you feel so powerless to impact your financial circumstances at this moment that it increases your stress to think about it? Then you would choose another life area on the Wheel to start with. For the sake of this example, I'm going to select one of my values, "connectedness," which has the potential to positively influence two or three life areas. What if you instituted a practice you associate strongly with "connectedness" such as, "Ask for help when I realize I need help?" Can you see that if you were to successfully establish that practice and receive the help you needed, that your sense of financial security—and peace of mind—could potentially increase, too? After all, financial security is ultimately about your ability to survive, which is much less about money than most of people think.

Take Action

Identify the new practice(s) and, if possible, assign a frequency to each one. For example, "Ask for help when I realize I need help" could be changed to "Check in with myself once a day. Ask 'Is there something I need help with today?' If yes, request it." (I have devoted an entire step to asking for help. If you read this example and cringed, make sure to read Step 4.)

GIFTS, TALENTS, AND BUSINESS ACTIVITIES

Keep away from people who try to belittle your ambitions. Small people always do that, but the really great make you feel that you, too, can become great.

—Mark Twain

Remembering, naming, and reclaiming your gifts and talents can be fun. It also has the potential to frustrate you, especially if you have veered off course from the hopes and dreams of your youth. If you discover that you have veered far off course, I ask that you trust in your ability to change. You have everything you need in you to uncover, reclaim, and use your unique gifts.

What makes it so difficult to see your gifts and talents as gifts and talents? We are a bit crazy. We think that if something is easy for us that it is easy for everyone. Imagine, for a moment, that you are watching a fish swimming around in the sea. It is just doing its thing, using its fins to glide through the water, with its unique shape and color and maybe a few barnacles for decoration. You watch this fish and revel in its perfection. Now shift perspectives. Imagine that you are that fish. Can you see your exquisite, unique qualities? Do you notice how beautifully you move through the water, marveling at your ability to live, breathe, and thrive in that water 24 hours a day, 7 days a week? Do you appreciate your unique shape and admire your fish scales, cuts, scratches, and all? Probably not. But it does not mean that you, Mr. or Ms. Fish, are not remarkable. You just can't see it.

We are like the fish, with one potential advantage; we have mirrors. Unfortunately, most people look at their reflected images with distorted eyes, filtering their vision with a hugely skewed sense of what is actually in front of them. Furthermore, it is a superficial image, one that only shows your surface. It is nearly impossible to observe yourself as you move about your life, using those gifts and talents without one iota of conscious thought. In that way, you are exactly like the fish, glorious just because you exist, yet ignorant of your perfection, barnacles and all.

Going on a Talent Hunt

The questions that follow give you access to what you don't normally see. If they look familiar, and you have answered them before, I invite you to answer them again. I find that each time you answer questions like these you either deepen your appreciation of what you already know—and may have forgotten—or uncover yet another gift.

Unearth Your Unique Gifts—Self-Assessment

1. Why do people hire you?
   a. If you are a W-2 employee, think about your last two or three jobs. What do you think made you stand out from the crowd of other applicants?
   b. If you are self-employed or own a small business, why do you think you've been successful?
2. What do your friends and/or bosses or customers rely on you for? (If you normally dismiss compliments, now's the time to retrieve them from your memory.)
3. What business activities do you most enjoy doing?
4. What specific talents do you call upon in difficult situations?
5. What talents do you wish you could use in your business, or at work, more than you do now?

Your answers to the five questions hold important clues to your success and sense of satisfaction. One client said that when she summarized her answers to these questions she uncovered her personal mission statement, a surprising and empowering result.

Guiding Notes

1. As simple as the above questions appear, you may find that some questions will be easier to answer than others. All 5 questions point to the same set of talents and abilities, just from different angles. If you find yourself stumped by one question, go to another that's easier to answer. Then go back.
2. Remember that you are like the fish. It's not easy to see yourself the way others see you. If you tend to discount your talents as boring, normal or dull, use whatever techniques you know to help get you out of your critical, left-brain thinking. Try using one of the tools introduced in the beginning of this chapter to help unlock your creativity and quiet your mind. Let the words flow. Don't edit or censor your responses, and don't worry if your answers don't seem to make sense.
3. Do your best to answer all the questions. If you feel resistance or confusion, put the questions aside and come back to them again at another time. Sometimes it helps to change your location to get a different perspective.
4. If you're an extrovert and are better able to hear your thoughts in conversation with someone else, find someone to ask you the questions and to take notes or record your replies. Be sure to ask them to let your thoughts guide the conversation. They may want to help you answer the questions—and you may want them to—but it's important at this juncture in the process that *you* start to see *you*.

After answering the questions on your own, ask a trusted friend or family member—or talk to your coach—about what you're uncovering through your replies. (Leave those who tend to be critical out of this!) Ask him or her to review what you've come up with. Ask if you seem to be missing anything, or if they see something you have not. Study your replies more than once. Circle or highlight words that seem important. Look for repeating themes.

Again, take note if you are judging yourself or if you feel bored by what you see. If you find yourself thinking that nothing you've got here is all that special or new or surprising, just notice the judgment but don't make any decisions just yet.

Carry It Forward

Why have I asked you to take this time to map out your "perfect life," identify your role models, confirm your values and uncover your unique, life-giving talents? What does this have to do with your business or career, and your recovery? Because you can't—and don't have to—return to business with the same set of unconscious, driven behaviors as before. This is the message Nedi took to heart when she attended my workshop after having spent the previous six years in bed. Everything you do, from now on, has the potential to rebuild or weaken. I know that sounds severe, but I say this with love and compassion. Remember, my own comeback story took 13 years.

Armed with a bag full of new awareness, you are now in a position to reconstruct your business or career in such a way that has the potential to replenish, nurture, succeed and grow. You're ready for Step 3: Back to Business Under "New Management."

5 Things to Remember, to Try, and to Discard

5 Things to Remember

1. A genie in a different bottle is still a genie
2. This is a perfect time to revisit forgotten dreams
3. You have the right to dream outside the box
4. You're as unique and perfect as "the fish"
5. You can't appreciate in someone else a quality you don't have access to yourself

5 Things to Try

1. Buy a set of colored pens or pencils and play around with construction paper
2. Start 2 new practices that increase alignment with your values
3. Allocate one more hour per day to a business activity you love
4. List 5 new ways you can use your gifts to make money
5. Interview or research the life of someone you admire

5 Things to Discard

1. Goals that don't match your values
2. Any and all efforts to be someone other than yourself
3. One project or commitment that you absolutely hate
4. Work without play
5. Belief in feedback delivered by naysayers

Step 3:
Back to Business Under "New Management"

Happiness is when what you think, what you say and what you do are in harmony.

—Mohandas Gandhi

The first two steps of the comeback plan directed you to look inside, to put your needs, desires, and wants front and center. Now that you are armed with this information, Step 3: Back to Business Under "New Management," will guide you back to work, with your attention facing outward, towards "real world" concerns: How will you rebuild your business or career with the least amount of unnecessary effort, and where should you begin? Your blueprint for success will account for your personal wellness plan, increasing the likelihood that your comeback plan will succeed. As you move away from internal exploration and start making decisions that will direct your external actions, I encourage you to keep your responses to the exercises in the first two chapters close at hand.

I'll start by outlining the questions that are likely to arise when you put your attention on getting out of bed and back to business.

They are big questions, so don't be concerned if you can't answer them thoroughly right now. You'll have plenty of opportunity to answer them more thoroughly as you read and do the exercises in this chapter. To get started, gauge your initial responses to the "First Impression" questions that follow, as your gut reactions are important.

First Impressions—What Will You Do Now?

1. Do you think you will go back to the same business, job, or career?

If you answered "yes":

2. What, if anything, needs to change?
3. Can you rebuild your business using the same business model as before, or do you need to change the model in order to increase your leverage and have more flexibility?

If you answered "no" to question number 1:

4. What do you think you'd like to do, instead?
5. What existing skills, tools, and resources would you most like to carry forward into the new business, job, or career?

Either way:

6. What tools or new skills do you need to acquire or learn?
7. What kind of help do you need? From whom?
8. How much energy and time do you personally have to run and manage your business (or do your job) on an average day right now?

Keep your responses to these questions in mind as you continue reading. The rest of the chapter will help you verify or modify your initial responses with practical considerations.

SIX FOUNDATIONAL BUSINESS QUESTIONS

Every business—your own, or the one you work for—is built around the responses to six basic questions. If you are an established business owner, you have probably answered them at least once—when you started the business—if not once a year. No business is a stagnant, unchanging organism. It can't be if it is to grow and thrive. Furthermore, entrepreneurs themselves evolve and grow. Priorities, needs, and goals change. Yours certainly have. This is the perfect time to revisit the six foundational business questions, which we will answer together in this chapter.

1. Why did you choose this business or line of work?
2. Who do you or the business serve?
3. What do you or the business do for the people or organizations it serves?
4. How and where does the work get done?
5. Who does the work?
6. How do you or the business make money?

They are only six questions but their answers are as varied and as unique as the people who own, manage, and run a business. The possibilities are infinite and *there is no single formula for success.* The fact that there is no one formula for success can be good news or bad news, depending on how you look at it. I have seen too many people (including myself) try to copy someone else's formula for success, only to find themselves out hundreds or thousands of dollars and sorely disappointed with the results. Therefore, I believe that *the fact that there is no single formula for success is good news.*

Remember, this is *your* comeback story. You may need to learn new skills or take some classes in order to upgrade your approach, or revisit some operating assumptions you made before you became ill. That is to be expected. However, there's is a qualitative difference between looking for "the answer" and learning something that will help you do your work more effectively or make better decisions. Knowledge improves wisdom. In the end, though, you must decide how and what your business or career will be.

If you are thinking about starting a business instead of going back to a job, I strongly encourage you to take all the time needed to review the information in Step 3. If you are returning to a job, you too will benefit from thinking about these questions because the organization you work for must address them. This is a perfect opportunity to think about what kind of organization you want to work for, how you want to work, and how you want to make your money. Where needed, I have added specific guidance to help you resurrect your career "under new management."

Why Did You Choose This Business or Line of Work?

"Why" comes before anything else. Knowing "why?" you do what you do will help keep you grounded and motivated when things become difficult. It will improve your ability to wade through the multitude of opportunities that come your way, to choose the ones that serve your purpose and ignore the ones that do not. When your energy is particularly low and you are in pain, remembering why you're doing something can guide you towards action that lifts your energy.

"Why?" will incorporate your purpose, your calling, your goals, and your personal priorities. Your personal priorities will reflect your values, your lifestyle needs, and your personal motivations. Many successful enterprises were initially launched in response to a spark of an idea that addressed the founder's frustration, pain, or passion. Others were launched in response to a perceived need that the owner believed he or she could successfully address. Here are several examples of generic "whys":

1. Something undesired happened to me; I don't want it to happen to you.
2. I figured out how to deal with something. I'm excited to share it with the world.
3. I dreamed of such-and-such but couldn't find it, so I built it myself.
4. I love so-and-so and could do it or talk about it all day long. The business gives me a way to do just that.

5. I want a business (or job) that will give me a lot of personal freedom, the ability to make decent money, and use my talents most effectively.

Through significant dietary and lifestyle changes, within six months of being diagnosed with Multiple Sclerosis, Laurie Erdman was able to put her symptoms into remission. Her experience was so dramatic that she found herself inspired to start a business helping others do the same. Her "why" falls under motivations 2 and 5.

The moment that sticks with me was about two months after I was diagnosed. I was having dinner with a friend. We were having a stream of consciousness conversation about the question of life. I said, "I don't know what I'm doing here," and she asked me "What would your ideal day look like?" At that point I knew that I didn't want to go to an office every day. I wanted to do something where there would be much more variety in my day. Clearly, it would be through self-employment but I didn't know what I'd be doing... I thought about being a yoga instructor. I was also creating a lot of pottery, which was very therapeutic, and I thought it might be that.

It seemed that every time I turned around I kept running into a "life coach." I was fascinated with their lifestyle: They were speaking, they were seeing clients...I loved the flexibility in their day. But I didn't want to be a life coach. I didn't want to do that. I remember having conversations with my husband, telling him that I thought this was interesting but not something I thought I wanted to do. And then the next day, I'd run into another [life coach]! And I thought "Oh my God." So I decided to do some research. One day I was online (I think I was looking at Wikipedia), and they listed different kinds of coaches. So I was scrolling through and then I saw the words "health coach."

This was around the 5-month mark [after my diagnosis] and I was already starting to see profound changes in my body. Having gone through some pretty tough challenges—making difficult dietary and lifestyle changes, putting me first, and things like that—I was starting to figure things out. That was about the time that I came across those words [health coach]. I thought, "Okay, I've been on the journey, I've been through the dark place. This is my opportunity to go back to the tribe and share something." Of course, this was still really early on, but that was the moment. I went searching from there and then found a [health coach training] program.

When you read Laurie's account of her "aha" moment, did you notice that she did not get the answer right away? She kept asking the questions until "it" clicked in. Whatever you do, don't give up. Trust that your answers will come at just the right time.

Self-Discovery

Write a short paragraph (2 or 3 sentences maximum) that summarizes why you want to go back to work, to your existing business, a new business or your job. It may help to review your responses to the exercises in Step 2, paying special attention to your values, perfect-day and perfect-work scenarios, and the gifts you identified in the talent hunt.

Who Do You or the Business Serve?

After "why," "who" is the single most important question that must be answered if you are to build or be a part of a business that will draw *you* into its service every day you wake up to work. It doesn't matter if you're talking about improving business systems, developing a better car or tending to the welfare of the environment, all businesses are designed to offer a solution to a perceived problem that ultimately benefits either people or other living organisms. Test it out. Company problems are people problems. Financial problems are people problems. Environmental problems are living, breathing creature problems. Animal rights issues are planetary and people-driven concerns.

The best business or organization for you will serve a group of people or a cause that you care about. Numerous studies have found that people perform better when the solution or service taps into a problem, need, or want they believe in and care about. If your work is to be more than a way to pay the bills, it has to be meaningful—for you—and offer you a sense of personal satisfaction and accomplishment. Teresa Amabile, a professor at Harvard Business School, and Steven Kramer, an independent researcher, the authors of *"The Progress Principle,"* collected nearly 12,000 electronic diary entries from 238 professionals in seven different companies.[1] They observed that:

- Employees are far more likely to have new ideas on days when they feel happier.
- Workers perform better when they are happily engaged in what they do.
- As long as workers experience their labor as meaningful, progress is often followed by joy and excitement about the work.

Their conclusions seem obvious, yet so many people get stuck in businesses or jobs that don't feed their souls, and stay in them out of survival until some life event knocks them out of complacency.

Identifying "who" you or your business serves is not only important for your own sense of fulfillment, it's critically important to your marketing efforts. For now, I'd like you to think about who (or what) you feel a strong connection to or passion about. (If you work for a company, you can answer the "who?" questions, too. There's no reason that your work life can't be as energizing and fulfilling as that of an entrepreneur.)

For Your Consideration

1. Who, or what cause(s), do you care about?
2. Who in your life do you most enjoy spending time with?
3. What do you most like about them?
4. What do they care about?

(continued)

5. How do you feel when you're around them?
6. What kinds of stories move you?
7. Who has come to you for help? What do they ask you to help them with?
8. What kinds of people would you most like to work with? What are they like?

Summarize Your Findings: I recommend you take a break—for at least two hours, if not an entire day—so that your unconscious mind can go to work on your replies to the questions above before answering the next three questions. When you come back, review your answers to the questions above:

1. How would you summarize your ideal work?
2. Who or what do you, or does the business, serve when doing that work?
3. How would you describe the kind of people you would most enjoy working with and/or for?

What Do You or the Business Do for the People or Organizations It Serves?

When you ask someone what they do, they'll often tell you their job title or function: I am the CEO of XYZ Company, I am a wellness coach, I am an IT consultant, I am a human resources manager, etc. While these are apt descriptions of a job title or business function, they are inadequate descriptions of "what" a person or company actually does, and they leave a lot of room for interpretation. Think about the IT consultant. There are a number of different services that they could offer.

- They could specialize in keeping home-based business computers free from virus threats.
- They could specialize in coordinating complex installations of integrated telephone and computer systems in Fortune 500 companies.
- They could help government agencies stay up-to-date with their data management software systems.

■ They could be Apple consultants that help retail operations install and customize point-of-sale (cash register) systems using Apple's proprietary software.

Those are just four examples that popped into my head about "what" an IT consultant or consulting firm might do. Did you notice that embedded in my sample "what" statements I also mentioned who they do it for (home-based businesses, Fortune 500 companies, government agencies and retail operations using Apple's proprietary point-of-sale software)? It's hard to separate "who" from "what," which is why I have encouraged you to first identify "who" the business serves.

Go back to your responses to the eight questions about whom, or what cause, you're most interested in and use the questions below to brainstorm ideas about "what" your company could do to improve their businesses or lives. Even if you are rebuilding an existing business, it's a worthwhile exercise.

For Your Consideration

1. List three to five typical needs of your target customer/client/ cause/employer.
2. For each need, name one to three ways you help them (or could help them) resolve their issues.
3. Review your responses to questions 1 and 2, and develop three to five short sentences that describe how they feel or what they experience after they use your product or service, or hire you.[2] For example:
   - After business owners work with us, their desk tops are so well organized that they feel like they just got back three hours of sunlight every day.
   - After women try our targeted nutritional program, they feel at least 10 years younger. Their energy is up and their need for sleep is down.

(continued)

- After a company hires me to oversee their social media cam-
  paigns they exceed sales projections. They wonder how they
  got along without me.
4. Develop two or three short summary statements about who you
  or your business serves and what you offer.

When the "what" is tied to a specific "who," your target customer—or employer—will feel that you know who they are, and you will, too. If you're having difficulties developing a short statement about your offer, go back to your "who." Either you're not yet specific enough or you have not connected to their needs.

How and Where Does the Work Get Done?

After you have (re)defined who you or your business serves and what it does for your "audience," you will be poised to (re)assess "how" you deliver the results. Table 3.1 presents a brief list of the most common business delivery systems. Each lends itself to a different management model and organizational structure. Some are location-dependent and others are not. Some can be conducted from the comfort of your home or bed, and others are best conducted in public locations.

As you review Table 3.1, first identify which of the four business types (retail, service, production, or education) best describes your current business, or the one you want to start or work for. Then look at the list of delivery systems in the right-hand column for your selected business type, and identify which ones you could employ to put your services or products in the hands of your clients/customers/employer. The delivery systems listed are not mutually exclusive. For example, a marketing consultant could sell information products through a website, or a local bakery could add an online order component to sell goods to customers in other

TABLE 3.1
Type of Business and Delivery Systems

Type of Business	Delivery System
Retail	Online
	Offline (brick and mortar stores)
	Home parties
Services	One-on-one
	Group
	In-person
	Virtual (phone or online)
	For profit
	Non-profit
	Government
	Home-based
	Office/storefront location
Production	Manufacturer
	Distributor/importer
	Designer/inventor
	Wholesaler/broker
	Retailer/reseller (eBay, for example)
Education	Virtual (online or phone)
	Home-based
	Elementary/secondary schools
	Colleges/universities
	Independent learning centers

locations. As an employee, a university instructor could teach on-campus classes two days per week and distance learning classes the other three days.

Business owners who have experienced a devastating health setback report that if their business tanked while they were in the acute phase of their illness or injury, they came back to business with the realization that the old delivery model ("how") exposed them to too much financial risk, or was no longer feasible for other reasons. Business coach and professional speaker Susan Bock changed "how" she delivered her services after a rigorous physical therapy schedule, following shoulder surgery, took her out of commission for six months.

> My business crashed. It came to a screeching halt because I was my product and my service. Because I was so restricted in what I could do, what had been a reasonably comfortable annual income went into the toilet. For three months following surgery, I could not work at all. That may not sound like very long but if you don't get paid, it is significant. However, I can look back and say I am grateful for that whole experience because it required me to look at different business models. It provided me with an opportunity to become very creative, break some old moulds, let go of outdated beliefs, and create a business that was flexible and allowed me to do what I do best.

> Before my surgery, the model was one-on-one, in-person coaching. I preferred face-to-face coaching so I could take in the totality of the whole person. That was my choice. Occasionally my clients would come to me, but for the most part I would drive to their location, anywhere from San Diego to Santa Barbara. The new model is phone coaching, which has opened my services up to the whole world. Perhaps a more important component is that I developed self-directed learning products. I now have numerous products for sale on my website that can be purchased at any time. The products are self-directed, but if someone chooses to follow-up and buy coaching, they can do that.

Through these two changes, making herself available for coaching by telephone and creating a multitude of self-directed learning products for her client base, Susan has decreased her financial vulnerability in several ways: She widened her market base, created the potential for "passive revenue," and made it possible to continue offering personal service if she needs to "work from bed" in the future. Susan is a professional speaker, too. Her programs and products can be used as platforms for paid speaking engagements. They, in turn, give her more opportunities to sell her products and services. What's more, products are built around systems. Systems can be licensed to others or taught to others, so she could add other revenue streams in the future, assuming an ever-increasing demand for her various products and programs. Finally, through this multi-pronged business model, she will be in a much better position to sell the assets when she is ready to retire and/or move onto something else.

For Your Consideration

1. In light of what you know about your values, your perfect work environment, skills and talents, and the overall state of your health, which one or two business types and delivery systems are most attractive to you?
2. How could you change your business model to reduce financial vulnerability and increase your revenue opportunities?
3. If you work for a company, have these questions sparked some ideas about other avenues for employment?

Who Does the Work?

Some businesses, especially home-based businesses, are started by sole owners who assume virtually 100% of the responsibility for all business tasks. This is a time-consuming commitment for even the healthiest of entrepreneurs. It can be tremendously limiting for the entrepreneur who is not operating at 100% capacity.

Many people, whether healthy or not, choose the path of self-employment for several common reasons. Most of these reasons start with the word "freedom":

- Freedom to do work that matters
- Freedom to set your own hours
- Freedom to make more money for each hour you work
- Freedom to work in an environment that suits you best (even from bed)
- Freedom to grow at your own pace

- Freedom to do the kind of work you most enjoy
- Freedom to enjoy a full personal life

Yet, with no staff or outside assistance, obtaining and maintaining that freedom is tricky. You are the CEO, head of marketing and sales, administrative assistant, production team, R&D team, file clerk, bookkeeper, receptionist, and service provider. With you at the helm and having the sole responsibility for every aspect of running the business, *any level of success will start to eat away at several of these freedoms.*

Choosing the Best Role(s) for Yourself

As a coach, I have explored, at length, the importance of understanding the best use of your time and talents in service of the business. My interviews with independent business owners underscored just how critical it is to know which roles in the business are best for you, and how important it is to exert most (50% or more) of your personal time and energy towards those specific roles. It's good for your health and good for business.

Team sports offer a useful insight into the brilliance of putting the right people on the team in the right positions, or roles. All positions are needed to win the game, yet not all positions are the same. Positions (roles) are assigned according to each team member's greatest strengths. Furthermore, the more value someone offers to the position, or the more essential the position is to winning the game, the more money they typically earn.

The same is true in your business. Of course, when it is all on you, or you and just a few other people, you'll have to juggle the various roles. However, that doesn't automatically override the team analogy. As a matter of fact, if you add just one player to your business team—assuming you choose your person well and put them in the right position—the overall impact will be greater than one plus one. With the right person you get a thinking partner, you can stop handling tasks that slow you down—plus, they should be able to do it equally as fast, if not faster, than you—and you are less vulnerable to "a bad day."

The business owners I interviewed that had already built a small team fared better during the most acute phase of their illnesses than those who had not previously engaged a single person to help in their business. They reported that when their symptoms, and side effects of treatment, required that they cut back their working time by as much as 75 percent, their businesses remained afloat. Their personal revenue may have decreased because they could not carry their usual workload, but the business did not come to a screeching halt.

Professional writer Kristina Anderson worked as much as she could for as long as she could to fulfill existing contracts, even after she started chemotherapy treatments following a double mastectomy. But, when the side effects of treatment became too much and it took everything she had to "drag herself to her computer," she "called on the bank of editors and writers" she had already hired for earlier projects to do the work she could no longer do. Her personal income dropped by half because she had to pay the other writers, but the business stayed afloat.

Business coach and author C.J. Hayden reported that when she was hit with a disruptive digestive illness and persistent insomnia, she relied heavily on her team of two—a long-standing virtual assistant and a business development partner—to help keep her business afloat when she was personally limited to working just two hours a day. Her revenue decreased when her symptoms were at their worst because she could not personally work with the same number of clients as she normally did, and she had to stop accepting speaking engagements and writing assignments for a few months. However, the business, as a whole, was not significantly impacted. Her two team members were able to field calls and emails, answer customer inquiries, fulfill orders, help with sales and marketing, and continue to keep things afloat.

To help you identify the best role(s) for you in your business (or the one you work for), I'll continue with the sports analogy and talk in terms of "hats" instead of positions. In place of terms like CEO, manager, customer service, etc. to describe the hats, I'll use role-oriented names for the hats and limit your choices to six:

- Visionary/Strategist
- Worker/Service Deliverer
- Promoter/Connector/Responder
- Developer/Inventor/Creator
- Organizer/Manager
- Administrative/Administrator

Each hat captures a range of talents, skills, tasks, and projects, as well as typical roles that are associated with the "nature" of each hat, as described below. This is by no means a complete list of all possible business roles, functions, and responsibilities. However, you should be able detect which hats (roles) are the best for you.

TABLE 3.2
Which Hat Fits Best?

Hat or Role	Associated Tasks or Functions	Response
Visionary/Strategist	*Big picture goals, strategy, and direction.* Often the face of the business. Keeps abreast of trends. Establishes and models vision, mission, and standards. Leader, thought leader. Keeper of the flame.	
Organizer/Manager	*Organizing or managing workflow, systems and/or people.* Responsible for execution and management of the vision and strategies. Forecasting and monitoring. P&L's, debit/credit management, inventory. Resource planning (human and physical).	

(Continued)

Hat or Role	Associated Tasks or Functions	Response
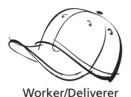 Worker/Deliverer	*Products, services, fulfillment.* Performs the core work of the business. Manufactures products, delivers services, engages with customers to fulfill requests, take orders or resolve problems.	
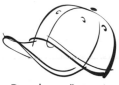 Developer/Inventor	*Developing, creating, inventing or designing products, services, materials, and/or solutions.* Inventing and creating new offerings. Designs products, programs, and marketing tools. Research, writing, curriculum, upgrades, improvements and innovations.	
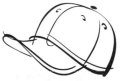 Promoter/Connector/ Responder	*Marketing and sales online and offline, customer relationship management.* Lead generation, networking, cold/warm calls, email campaigns, alliance strategies, public speaking, writing, publicity, web promotion, and/or social media. Responds to inquiries, makes sales presentations and closes deals.	
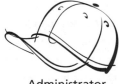 Administrator	*Filing, financials, word processing, and other support functions.* Editing, proofing, organizing email, reception/phone calls, web site maintenance, computer care and updates, accounts payable and receivables, shopping cart and accounting systems, etc.	

Try This on for Size

1. Read the short list of tasks and areas of responsibility associated with each hat in Table 3.2. As you're reviewing the lists, imagine that you're trying each hat on. Notice your immediate response. Do you feel energized and happy, or annoyed and frustrated? (As always, try to keep your mind out of it. Remember, your body is your guide now.)
2. Next, imagine that you set off to work and that you get to (or have to) wear only one hat for an entire day. Which hat(s) would you happily wear most often if time, money, or health were not a concern?
3. Once you try each hat on, even if only in your imagination, use the following symbols to signify your response to each of the hats. If there are some tasks or areas of responsibility that you do enjoy within a hat category that feels otherwise, repugnant, feel free to make note of it, but don't change your overall feeling associated with that hat.

    ♥–Love it, fully engages my key talents and skills, *and* is great for the business.

    ★–Uses my skills and some of my natural talent but is not quite as useful in light of my available time and energy.

    ⇓–Ugh, if I never have to do this again life would be great. It may be good for the business but it is not good for me!
4. Note your responses in the "Response" column of Table 3.2 or in your program notebook.

The hats you would happily wear all day long will become obvious. Those hats (roles) for which you have a natural affinity will cause a spontaneous smile to bloom on your face and a deepening of your breath, perhaps even a sigh of relief. You might even notice your heart center open up with a sense of joy. The hats you'd be happy to never wear again will cause you to retract, perhaps with a groan or a closed off feeling. You might even feel disgusted or mildly depressed.

Admittedly, no matter which hats you are most drawn to wearing, it's unlikely that you'll wear only one hat on any given day. Such is business life. Nonetheless, by knowing which business roles are most fun, interesting, and energizing, you can make better strategic decisions about the best use of your time and energy in service of your goals. Additionally—this is where it gets exciting—you will be able to make better decisions about what kind of help you need. In Step 6, "Build Capacity, Organize for Success," I'll show you how to use this information to develop a "master planning schedule" that will enable you to plan your business life to take advantage of your preferred roles, talents, and strengths.

Your Essential Business Role(s)

Engaging in work that leverages your "essential business roles," represented by the two or three hats that fit best can (1) improve your business outcomes and (2) increase your sense of personal satisfaction. Furthermore:

- Work will feel less like work and more like play.
- You can work fewer hours in the day (because you are more effective and focused).
- You can reasonably expect to finish the projects that matter most in less time.
- You will be able to identify who you must hire or delegate to in order to stay focused on the tasks associated with the roles and tasks that are best for you and for the business.

I once led a workshop for a group of women business owners, "Managing the Business Hats." When giving instructions about how to do the exercise I outlined above, and I put on the "Promoter" hat, I blurted out, "I hate this hat." Although my statement was infused with energy, it was a simple statement of fact. At that point, I had not yet bundled "connecter" with "promoter," which I now see as the flip side of the same business function. I am a good connector but I am not a good self-promoter. My business—and I—had been suffering as a result. I resolved right then and there to find someone who could take on most of the promotional aspects of running my business so that my message could get out to the people I wanted to reach, without undue interference from a personal "ugh!" factor. This allowed me to stay focused on my strengths (writing, developing, connecting), making me a much happier, healthier, and more effective business owner.

I didn't look for help right away, and when I did it took me several months to find the right people to add to my team. I knew I found the right marketing assistant when another coach forwarded an email announcing an opportunity to be interviewed on an internet radio show. I wanted to pursue the opportunity but I did not want to write and send the pitch myself. I was delighted to discover that my new marketing assistant was well equipped with just the right skills. When I read what she prepared, it was different than anything I would have done.

I asked my new assistant to review lists she already subscribed to for other similar opportunities. I could have subscribed to them, myself, but I knew I would not be consistent with my efforts. After only three pitches we landed the first interview. If she had not been reviewing the daily distribution of new opportunities I'd never have seen the others. If I had seen them, the likelihood that I'd pitch myself was about 5 percent, on a good day. It took a few more months to find the other essential team member, a strategic marketing consultant with talent for big-picture planning and promotion. How do you spell relief? D-e-l-e-g-a-t-i-o-n!

Summarize Your Findings

Based on your assessment of which hats fit best, what kinds of changes do you need to make so that you can wear those hats more often, and get rid of the "ugh" hats entirely?

Keep this information on hand. You'll refer back to it again in Step 4: "Recruit and Request—Ask for Help," and in Step 6, "Build Capacity, Organize for Success."

How Do You or the Business Make Money?

*When your income is insufficient to meet the most basic
of financial needs, it creates a chronic condition much like
undernourishment does.*

—Joan Friedlander

This is where the rubber meets the road. No matter how great your idea or how much fun you're having, if your business does not generate the revenue needed to keep it up and running, or you're not getting paid enough to meet your expenses, it's ultimately unsustainable. The revenue models for service-based businesses are different than the models for product-based businesses. The overhead and potential profitability for each (gross sales minus all business expenses) differs greatly, too. To remain within the scope of this book, I'll only outline various revenue models that are associated with businesses you can most easily run or work for from your home, or bed. I will not discuss the additional complexities associated with external product development and manufacturing, such as inventory management, production issues and overhead costs.

The following are examples of viable revenue models for a variety of businesses. Most of the specific examples given to illustrate each model can be executed or managed from the comfort of your home or bed. Many can be done on a limited basis if you can only work a few hours a day. If you are not returning to or starting a business, but are returning to a new or former job, you'll find a list of "revenue models" for employees following the "Revenue Models for Business Owners."

Revenue Models for Business Owners

Fee for Service Models

Hourly Fee—Charging clients by the hour (or some other benchmark, like "per page") is a common business practice among consultants and other service providers such as graphic designers, editors, virtual assistants, fee-only financial planners, coaches, etc. It is certainly a reasonable option, and expected by many clients. Examples:

- Financial planner charges $175/hour for a 2-hour financial review to attract clients who may be reluctant to commit to higher-priced services up front
- Freelance editor charges $10/page, knowing that she can usually review 5 pages in an hour

Many professional service providers discover that charging by the hour is not always the most profitable approach. Prospects and clients are inclined to put their attention on how much you're making per hour instead of the results, value, and experience they receive from using your services or products. You may do that, too. If the traditional fees associated with your profession are more than you feel comfortable charging, you may short-change yourself by giving time away or undercutting your fees. What's more, when you charge per billable hour, you may neglect to make it a point to understand the real value of your customers' investments in your services. If your work (services or products) saves people or companies time, waste, or money, the real value to them can be tremendous, many more times than what you're charging them per hour.

If it is best for you, either because of industry tradition or personal ease, to charge by the hour, I do not mean to suggest that you should stop doing so. As I said when I opened this chapter, the best business decisions are made when you know what works best for you at this moment in time. Furthermore, when making decisions about what you will charge for your products or services, it's often easiest to decide using money-per-hour calculations. Because your time and energy, and the value you offer, are all important elements in the revenue puzzle, I want you to have access to as much information as possible to put together a meaningful business that has the greatest potential to support you, on all levels.

C.J. Hayden outlined alternatives to the "hourly fee" revenue model in her article, "Entrepreneur on a Mission: What's Your Business Model?"[3] Where I have inserted my ideas and comments I used *italics*.

Day Rate—Instead of charging by the hour, you can charge by the day or half-day. This imposes a minimum on your clients, avoiding short appointments that fragment your work schedule. Examples:

- *Wardrobe consultant offers half-day virtual closet-clearing sessions for stay-at-home moms*
- Environmental market researcher conducting focus groups
- Massage therapist providing on-site massage for organizations

Project Fee—Charging a flat fee for each project allows you to bill for time you spend planning, researching, or just thinking about your client's issues. Clients often prefer flat fees because they can budget their funds more accurately. (*Your ability to accurately estimate the time required for planning, researching, or just thinking, will help you charge enough to meet your bottom-line requirements. To make sure you're charging enough, keep close track of your hours for the first few projects.*) Examples:

- Sustainability consulting firm advising clients on implementing responsible practices
- Psychologist offering psychological testing and assessment

Monthly Retainer—When you ask clients to pay by the month in advance, you can charge for your availability, not just service delivered. Your retainer can guarantee you a fixed number of hours (*and revenue*). If the client uses less, you still get paid. If they use more, you can charge extra. (*Be sure to outline the expectations in a contract.*)

- Recovery coach offering as-needed calls and e-mails in between sessions
- Political consultant providing ongoing campaign management and advice

Subcontractors/Employees—You can hire or contract with other professionals and have them deliver services on behalf of your company. These may be people who come to you with appropriate skills and experience already, or people you train to use your approach. Clients pay your company for these services and you keep a percentage for yourself. (*This can be especially appealing if your personal time and energy are limited, and you have developed a proprietary product or system.*)

■ Learning center with multiple teachers on staff (*online or on-site*)
■ Diversity training firm with trainers in multiple locations

Product- or Process-Based Models

Flat Fee—A wide variety of items can be sold for a flat fee to increase revenue for your enterprise. *"Services" can be packaged and sold to individuals or groups.* "Products" can also include services delivered in a defined package. Your buyers may be either existing clients, or others who can't afford to hire you individually. *Packaged services and products can take many forms, including but not limited to e-books, e-courses, self-study workbooks, group telephone seminars or webinars, etc.* Examples:

■ Cause marketing consultant packaging her wisdom in a do-it-yourself kit
■ Mediator offering public conflict resolution seminars (or webinars)

Subscription/Membership—Providing products or services by subscription, or memberships in your community, can provide a steady source of income and reduce marketing time. A sale made only once can continue to provide revenue.

■ Youth leadership trainer selling an educational CD series by monthly subscription
■ Nurse consultant hosting an online community for people with chronic illness
■ *Published authors joining together to offer other writers support through online coaching and limited editorial review*

Back-End Sales—Also called the "bait and hook" or "razor and blades" model, where you sell a product or service that requires periodic updates at an additional cost.

- Vegan weight loss expert offering frozen packaged meals delivered monthly
- Database of sustainable ingredients for cosmetics requiring quarterly updates

Licensing/Franchising—Packaging your approach so that others can replicate it with their own clients or in different locations. Your licensees or franchisees pay you a start-up fee to acquire your package, which may also include training. You may also offer them ongoing training and support in return for an annual renewal fee or a percentage of their earnings.

- Social enterprise employing homeless workers offers their model to other cities
- Trauma recovery therapist certifies other therapists in his/her approach

As Hayden said, "Any one of these models can be used to build an entire business, or you can combine different models together. For example, a consultant could charge a flat fee for assessments, then a day rate to deliver services. A coach could charge a subscription fee for group clients and a monthly retainer for clients worked with individually."

For Your Consideration

1. If you are rebuilding an existing business, ask yourself the following questions regarding your current revenue model.
   a. Is it sustainable going forward?
   b. If it's not sustainable, which model or models would be better?
   c. What else do you need to know? Who can you ask? Who in your industry is using a model you'd like to learn more about?

(continued)

2. If you are just starting a new business, or are thinking about starting one, which revenue model or models are most interesting
   to you?
   a. What questions do you have?
   b. What else do you need to know?
   c. Who can you ask for help?

Revenue Models for Employees

You may prefer to work for a business or organization as an
employee because you don't want to be responsible for marketing
and sales, because you do better with more structure and camaraderie, or you feel more comfortable with a reliable income base
and employee benefits. Employees have several "revenue" models to choose from as well. Just as for self-employed people and
small business owners, a job that is too demanding, physically
and financially, may be okay for a little while, but not forever. This
might be a good time to consider alternative revenue models or a
new job!

I got a big wake-up call in 1998—six years after my Crohn's
diagnosis—when my body sent me clues through a strange
infection in my right foot, not once but twice! Two unexplained
spontaneous abscesses in my right foot put me out of operating commission for a total of 14 weeks, 8 weeks in the summer months and 6 weeks in late fall. At that time I was the sole
employee of a career search firm, making less money than I
needed, and below my true earning capacity in light of my skill
set and experiences. Furthermore, I was doing work that was
adjacent to the work I wanted to do, but not "it" at all. There
was an implied promise that I would be able to coach some of
our clients that never materialized. Working alongside the business owner was not always easy, either, as he was rather intense
at times. (He used to pound on the keyboard when his computer

would freeze. I get it, it's frustrating, but pounding just didn't help! Plus, we worked in a small office with no visual or sound barriers between us.)

Recovering from surgery after a foot abscess was a lot easier than dealing with Crohn's flare-ups. Even though it was uncomfortable and inconvenient—I had to crawl up stairs to the doctor's office, hobble around on crutches, and I could not drive myself anywhere—it was a finite situation. However, when it happened the second time in one year, I had to ask myself, "What is going on here?" In one of those still and quiet moments, the answer came streaming through with the usual understated ease of most "divinely" delivered messages: "I don't have a leg to stand on."

That got my attention! It was time to extract myself from that job, to start making enough money to comfortably support myself and my son, and get started in earnest towards the profession that had been calling to me for the previous three years: coaching. Within just a few days of my revelation I gave notice, made an appointment to meet with a placement counselor at the local temp agency, and by the end of December had secured a "temp-to-perm" assignment with a benefits broker company. The position was easy to manage: It paid me more than I had made in any previous job, was only 1.5 miles from home, and the hours were reliably excellent. I was able to leave the office at 5:00 PM most days, a very good thing for a single mom of a 14-year-old. Because the job wasn't taxing financially, mentally, or emotionally, I had time and energy in the evening hours to start to construct the framework for my coaching business. Even if that had not been my goal, by paying attention to my body cues, I quickly made changes to improve my revenue position. Plus, the people I worked with at my new job were smart, fun, and sane.

The following are four common "revenue models" for employees. As you read through them, ask yourself, "Which of the four financial arrangements would be most supportive of my health and financial well-being now?" The examples are hardly representative of the many positions that you could find for each type of arrangement. You may want to research income models for your chosen field and ideal positions, or explore opportunities for employment associated with a salary structure that interests you.

Non-Exempt Hourly Wage—You're paid for the number of hours you work, and receive overtime pay (1.5 to 2 times your base hourly wage) when you work more than 40 hours per week, and on holidays. In some states, you also receive overtime wages when you work more than 8 hours a day. The following are two examples of this kind of situation:

- A full-time retail employee earning $10.00 per hour receives $15.00 per hour for overtime hours worked. The company offers benefits when an employee works more than 30 hours a week.
- A technical account manager earning $25.00 per hour is able to work from home two days a week. Overtime hours are limited and her base salary is more than enough.

Exempt Salary—Your pay is based on an hourly wage. However, your monthly earnings are calculated based on your annual income. You are paid the same amount every pay period no matter how many hours you work. Exempt employees sometimes receive quarterly or annual bonuses based on individual, team and/or company performance. Exempt employees are often referred to as being "on salary." Examples:

- A retail store manager earning $80,000 a year receives quarterly sales or performance bonuses. Actual number of hours worked varies by season and is highly dependent on one's time management and delegation skills.
- An executive in charge of sales and marketing has a base salary of $150,000 per year and earns bonuses based on team performance, plus trips and bonuses awarded in sales competitions. May be expected to work 50–70 hours per week.

Base Salary Plus Commission—You receive a base amount every pay period, and receive additional pay that is dependent on your performance. Your base salary may be less than others in comparable positions in different professions, or below your actual income needs. This is a typical arrangement in many sales-related positions. Examples:

- A sales engineer earning a substantial base salary receives a small percentage of total sales revenue.
- An account executive in an insurance company earning a reasonable base salary is additionally compensated through commissions or quarterly bonuses based on total team sales and renewals.

Commission Only—You receive a certain percentage of all sales you close, or have a part in closing. This is a typical arrangement in sales. Even though you work for a company, your income is dependent on you. The company usually receives a greater percentage of total revenue than you do. You might start out with a base salary plus commission arrangement, and "graduate" to commission-only after a pre-defined number of months. Examples:

- A personal investment consultant working for a large investment house receives 20% commission on all financial products purchased by clients he or she brings in, plus team bonuses. There is no ceiling on potential earnings but there are baseline measures that must be met to keep the position.
- An independent sales representative working for a start-up event production company earns 25% on all sales. He enjoys the flexible schedule and the thrill of being on the ground floor with a new company.

A Blended Option—Part-Time Subcontractor

This final option is more accurately represented as a self-employment option, but it can be viewed as a compromise opportunity, too. As a contractor or subcontractor you do not work for a company as a salaried employee but, instead, establish yourself as a specialized expert for a specific period of time at an agreed upon rate. The hourly or project rate is typically higher than if you were retained as employee.

Such opportunities often arise when a smaller company is in growth mode and does not have the capacity—or need—to pay a full-time salaried person to fulfill certain roles. They need a specialized expert relevant to a specific role, and who is available for a limited number of hours per week or a short time period to execute the work.

This kind of arrangement offers you revenue stability for the duration of the contract period. You will not receive health benefits, and when the contract ends you'll either need to seek renewal or find a new opportunity. Typically, an hourly or project rate is agreed upon and payment for services are billed monthly. Examples:

- A compensation consultant helps a business upgrade and manage salary and compensation packages for all levels of employees. He is kept on retainer for various associated projects for an agreed-upon period of time.
- A writer is retained to develop marketing and communications materials for a growing medical supply company. She oversees the development and revisions associated with all marketing materials, including web, print and internal communications.
- An executive coach works under the umbrella of a company that sells coaching services to government agencies. She receives payment at an agreed-upon rate for the hours she works directly with the client(s). She is not paid for the hours she puts in to prepare or follow up.

Summarize Your Thoughts

1. Which revenue/income model describes your current or most recent job position?
2. Knowing what you know now, is it still the best earning model for you?
3. If it's not, which other model would be better?
   a. What jobs came to mind when you read about your preferred revenue model? What positions might you qualify for?
   b. What concerns do you have about pursuing a new opportunity?
   c. What questions do you have and who can you ask?

THE ANSWER IS NOT ALWAYS EASY

You may discover that you need to change your employment situation because what you're doing now—or were doing before—is no longer a good fit. If the working conditions, the work, itself, the people and/or the income are not good for your health, you may find yourself compromising your values where you'd really rather not. Even when you do find a position that is much better for your health and well-being, you might still feel ambivalent. Audrey, who used to enjoy the prestige and earnings associated with a high-level management position in an exhilarating office environment, was often bored and frustrated by the same flexibility and understanding that helped her manage her health and well-being in her new job. She confessed that, though grateful for the flexibility, she would much rather do something that offered her greater mental stimulation, and a higher salary. She is attracted to business ownership, either as a replacement option or as a part-time evening endeavor, but she hesitates on two fronts:

- She is not confident that she has the capacity to add the tasks typically required to launch a new business to her existing schedule.
- She does not trust that she would make enough money to cover health insurance costs if she were to let go of her job and fly solo.

Hers are the questions and concerns that dominate the lives of people who live under the cloud of a chronic health problem and/or wavering levels of capacity on any given day. It can take months—or years—of trial and error before you find the right "formula" for you. Remember: *Circumstances change.* What you are required to do today may be different tomorrow. Present time and needs are just that. You are not stuck with decisions you make today if they do not suit you next year. Business or career success does not follow a straight-line trajectory, nor will you find "the formula" that will last a lifetime. Even McDonald's has had to evolve in response to pressures to add healthier options to their basic menu.

Armed with your gifts and talents, ideal life, values, and business model preferences, you are in an excellent position to make more informed, healthy decisions about how to rebuild or start anew. This is a good time to develop an action plan for reconstructing your business or career under "new management." Anytime you notice that you've gotten caught in a victim or blame cycle you can go back to Step 1, Beyond Survival, and select questions from "Dismantling the Comparison Trap" to dissolve your fear and false assumptions.

5 Things to Remember, Try, and Discard

5 Things to Remember

1. Your motivation for working (your "why?")
2. You can get back to meaningful work
3. This is your business/career, and no one else's
4. Pay attention to your body cues
5. You and your business—or organization you work for—perform better when you enjoy your work

5 Things to Try

1. Identify 5 ways you could make money serving people or a cause you care about
2. Explore alternative business models (or job opportunities)
3. Research a new business idea
4. Write a job description for your ideal hire (even if you don't plan to hire anyone)
5. Write your own comeback story as if it's already happened

5 Things to Discard

1. Someone else's dream for you
2. A job or business that doesn't sustain you
3. Must know now
4. Can't do it
5. "Hats" that don't fit

Step 4:
Recruit and Request—Ask for Help

It's not the load that breaks you down, it's the way you carry it.
—Lena Horne

YOU CAN'T DO IT ALONE ANYMORE—AND YOU DON'T HAVE TO

Entrepreneurs are, by nature, fairly independent people with a strong sense of capability and self-reliance. It's not surprising that the sudden dependency brought on by illness or injury is so devastating. Of course, sudden dependence—and its partner, unreliability—disturbs employees, too. I prided myself on being capable and reliable and felt horrible each time I had to take a disability leave. In my mind, my reputation as a "reliable worker" was in jeopardy. I felt guilty and embarrassed, not a pleasant combination.

You can try, but you cannot rebuild a business that is financially and physically sustainable by doing things the same way you've always done them. The rules have changed. Every person I interviewed mentioned just how difficult their new dependence was, at least initially. They also admitted that it was one of the gifts of their health crisis. Learning to ask for help changed their relationships—and their ability to recover—in positive ways. Yet, it's not as simple as just asking. There are important issues to consider: who can help, how they can help, as well as concerns about privacy or potential threats to the business (or your career) when word gets out, etc. These issues are addressed in Step 4 so that you can decide who can help and when.

Loss of self-reliance follows the same trajectory as the loss of a loved one. First there is denial, then there is anger, followed by bargaining and depression, and finally, acceptance. Interviews with a variety of business owners uncovered the following layers of acceptance, from somewhat passive acceptance to more proactive reliance.

- Admitting
- Accepting
- Allowing
- Asking

Admitting You Need Help

Admitting that something is awry can be an emotional and mental landmine. When I was about 7 years old I got sick on the playground at recess. I was mortified. I went back to the classroom, fully intending to keep quiet about it. Some boy in my class decided it was important to raise his hand and tell the teacher I'd thrown up. I suppose it's possible that he wanted to be helpful, but I felt like his purpose was to tattle on me and that I had done something wrong. Instead of steeping in quiet mortification by myself, my mishap became public knowledge. The teacher promptly sent me to the nurse's office.

The fear of being found out, of public humiliation and judgment, drives all of us to keep things hidden from ourselves first, and from others second. Of course, there's good reason to keep some things private. However, when you keep something hidden from your own view, either because you don't want to be hassled by the inconvenience or because you fear the worst, you risk a slower recovery. As Nedi, the songwriter, said when I asked what she wants people to know:

> I would tell them to reach out and ask for help. [I want them] to know they don't have to be alone or ashamed. Illness can make you feel cut off from the world because people don't understand your confusion … everybody is dealing with physical limitations, so we are really in the same boat. The more you ask for help, the less lonely you will be. And, I mean, not just the practical help of getting your shopping and laundry done. I really wished I would have asked my religious community to help. They could if I'd only asked … You can't ask for help if you won't admit you need it.

Accepting Temporary Dependence

Accepting that you need help is only possible after admitting that you are in trouble. Here's how Susan Bock described the transitions she went through, from sheer frustration to during her 6-month recovery from shoulder surgery.

> Following the surgery, for 6 months, 6 hours a day, I was hooked up to one of three different pieces of equipment. I was pretty confined as to what I could do, not just the activities but the timing within which I could do things because each of these 2 hour treatments had to be 2 hours apart. It was really a 12-hour day. Mentally, [the restrictions on my time] put me into a depressive state because I was incapable of doing what I had done previously. Being so restricted, unable to do as much, and having to accept that was a difficult process for me to go through. I didn't know I was going to have to be so dependent. For someone who prided herself for on being independent, it was a psychological drain equal to the physical challenges.

> **Question:** Did you get to a point of acceptance?

> Yes, the inner war was raging between my ego and intellect, which was very aware of what I should and shouldn't do. I'll say that the acceptance came first. I don't want to say I surrendered because to me that sounds like I gave in or gave up. I didn't. It was really about accepting that it is what it is. I needed to pace myself and accept

the fact that my body had to heal. I became the cheerleader of my recovery rather than the competitor who was interfering with it.

Allowing Others to Help

Allowing or permitting others to help you is the next step in opening up to receive help from others. I might have "allowed" that boy in my elementary school class to help me, but you can be sure I did not feel grateful for his unsolicited help. Allowing others to help you can be one of the more difficult acts of kindness towards yourself and towards others.

Susan helps us understand "allowing" through the continuation of her journey. I asked her when she was able to understand that the best road back to full recovery was through the path of acceptance. Just before she started to accept her situation, she allowed others to help her. Here is what she said.

> It was probably at the end of the second month when I said to my husband, "I need a break." I had to get out [of the house] because I was so confined. I visited my parents in Colorado. I guess by saying that it was okay to admit that I needed something other than what I was giving myself—whether that was love and attention or being in a different environment. By taking that trip and acknowledging that I needed to [give this] gift to myself to facilitate my recovery, is when the shift occurred. And, of course, I had to take the [physical therapy] equipment with me. My father is incredibly talented at building things and he replicated the "torture chair." I was very humbled by my parents' attention, and I felt their love. Yes, love is a powerful healing tool!

Allowing is all about receiving. If you are used to being the person that people come to for help or guidance, allowing others to help you, instead, will be uncomfortable. Being in the helping position may give you a sense of control, creating an invisible barrier of sorts, and is a way to keep the attention off of yourself and on others. When you are suddenly the one in need, it has the potential to create an emotional imbalance, and for you, the feeling of a loss of power. If you are usually "the giver" and you're feeling particularly unnerved by sudden dependency, I encourage you to ride with the feeling—to embrace your needs with humility—and allow others to help you. It has proven to be a transformational turning point for many who have traveled a similar road. It can forever change your relationship to your life, and to the people you care about most.

C.J. Hayden gained new appreciation for her friends and loved ones when she saw how readily they stepped in to help her during her six-month health ordeal. Here's what she said:

> I've become much more aware of the importance of having close relationships with friends and family because there were a lot of people in my personal life who were very supportive and helpful to me during that time period. It made me realize I [had been] putting more emphasis on my work and business than was healthy or appropriate, and that I should be spending more time with friends and family. I've made it a part of my weekly planning ritual to make sure that every week I'm doing something social or relationship oriented, and it's been wonderful. I've kept it up every week since I've started to recover, and I love it.

Accepting and allowing do not mean that you cannot refuse assistance. If the assistance being offered is not in your best interest and does not, in fact, help you, you are well within your right to respectfully decline or "negotiate" the offer and ask for something that is more helpful to you. However, there is a difference between respectfully declining specific assistance and refusing all offers of help. You can detect the difference through the degree of energy associated with your push-back. A stubborn refusal to accept assistance is not the same as a discerning response to the assistance being offered.

Asking for Help

Asking others for help is the last step on the continuum. Even when you do allow others in and accept offers of assistance, you may still hesitate to ask for help when you need it. Yet, your ability to ask for help gives you access to the kind of help you most need. While allowing and accepting assistance are positive steps in the right direction, asking others for help improves the likelihood that the kind of assistance you receive is the kind of assistance you need.

Self-Discovery

1. Where would you place yourself on the spectrum between admitting you need help and asking for help?
2. If you've hesitated to ask for help, or to accept offers of help, what has stopped you?

DUMP THE BURDEN MYTH

If you can't remember how to do the simplest of things, you need help. If you can't get around easily on your own, you still need help. If chemotherapy is making you sicker than a dog, you most definitely need help.

C.J. was used to relying on herself to track and manage her projects. When insomnia impacted her short-term memory, she was forced to change her approach. Here is how she described the experience.

If you can't sleep you lose your ability to remember, to process information, and your judgment becomes impaired. I had to learn to depend on other people, and on structures and mechanisms. Ordinarily, I rely on my brain a lot—I did not realize the extent to which I relied on my brain until I didn't have one. My to-do list is a prime example. I used to write a lot of things down, but I held a lot in my head, too. I was used to knowing what needs to be done without looking at a list. Because of the insomnia, it became necessary for me to keep detailed meticulous lists, and to ask people to help me remember things. There were times I'd space out just looking at the list.

I had to ask my virtual assistant to "poke" me when it was time for me to do certain things. I asked my life partner, Dave, to remind me about other things. I asked both of them to do some things for me that I would have usually done myself. I also asked my other team member, my business development person, to take more responsibility for things than I ordinarily would, and to remind me when things needed to be taken care of so that I would have a fall-back.

So, what would stop you from asking for help? Following are the three of the most common reasons given by my clients, either directly or in the unspoken:

- Misplaced identity
- Guilt
- Feeling Overwhelmed

Misplaced Identity

If you equate measurable output, productivity, and accomplishment with your value as a human being, you may find it particularly hard to adjust your thinking on this. But remember: You are a human being, with emphasis on "being." At a time like this, occasionally you must simply "be" and not "do." As a matter of fact, if you're at all like I was, your inability to *do* everything might just slow you down enough to *be* present for people in a way that you have not been for quite some time. If you are letting your entire identity rest on the fraction of it that relates to your work, you, my friend, have misplaced your identity.

We live in a busy, go-get-it world. A lot of people talk about how busy they are, insisting on the normalcy of a busy life. I have coached people who tell me that they have to do something productive every day—including both weekend days—and that if they are not productive they don't feel right inside. "I am busy" equals "I am successful." Socially, busyness is often equated with being popular or needed. This is such an extraordinarily sad state of affairs. Illness is one gigantic STOP sign. The body has to come back into balance. Doing, giving, getting, and achieving, are all reasonable aspects of the human experience, but not to the exclusion of the other side of the equation. Yang without Yin is unhealthy and ultimately, unreasonable.

I say these things as a perpetually recovering "Do-Bee"—someone who believes the best way to be successful is to take charge and get things done. Illness changed the dynamics between me and life. On those days when I was so sick that I had to stay in bed, I noticed a more loving, gentler version of myself emerge—I listened more and instructed less. My illness had temporarily removed the perpetual Ms. Busy Bossy Bee and replaced her with Ms. Present Calm Listening Bee! I don't know if my husband or son noticed the change, but I certainly did. I noticed the same shift in my manner when friends visited me in the hospital during that long 10-day stay. Without all the pressures associated with navigating "normal" life I became more centered and comfortable with myself, something that truly surprised me. I not only listened more, but the familiar fears and insecurities that accompanied daily living decreased significantly.

Guilt

No doubt, those who are closest to you will feel the "burden" of the extra assistance you require. The scales of give and take are out of balance. It's a fact. Yet, guilt, defined as "a feeling of responsibility or remorse for some offense, crime, wrong, etc., whether real or imagined,"[1] has the potential to cripple you and make it harder for everyone else. Stop for a moment. Think and question. Just what crime have you committed? Who have you offended? Are you really deserving of punishment (the consequences of a "guilty" verdict)? I doubt it, yet feelings of guilt are prevalent among those who are ill.

Debbie, whom you met in Step 2, was overcome by guilt when her illness made it extremely difficult to keep up with the responsibilities associated with running a research lab at a prestigious university. Her many responsibilities included assisting the students in preparing research papers for submission to scientific journals. Competition in the scientific community is fierce and the prestige of being published is high. When she hired me as her coach, it was to help her be more productive with her time, and to create a schedule for her work that would enable her to focus on what was really important, with a high priority placed on reviewing and submitting manuscripts.

Unfortunately, the reality of Debbie's illness was such that the details associated with this kind of work were simply more than she could handle. It took months before Debbie was able to admit to herself that she could no longer do this work. It was probably one of the most difficult things to accept, as she associated her incapacity with a strong sense of personal failure. Eventually, she was able to let go of her expectations and make her health a priority, thus deciding to take a disability leave. Once she was able to accept her situation, to accept the "help" that long-term disability insurance afforded her, it set her on a course of healing and self-discovery.

Guilty or Not?

If you are inclined to feel chronically guilty, see if you can release it through honest replies to the following questions.

1. Have you committed a punishable crime against someone?
2. Are you making unreasonable demands in light of your current situation?
3. In the big picture of things have you caused harm or offense to someone in your life?
4. Are you ultimately responsible for the health, well-being, and happiness of all people in your life?

The fourth question is a tricky one. You may feel that you have let people down. It might even be true. It is reasonable to feel badly when something that happens in your life causes discomfort or disappoints someone else. It is not reasonable to assume that said discomfort or disappointment permanently ruins their lives. We all experience, or ignite, disruptive events throughout our lives—you're in the midst of one now! Time and hindsight often reveal the gift or opportunity that may not have materialized without said disruption.

If you have been less than gracious in your relationships of late, then regret, disguised as guilt, would be a reasonable temporary response. If that's the case, then you only need to acknowledge your missteps to anyone who has been affected and adjust your behavior or attitude. Once the source of the guilt is discovered, holding on to it helps no one. Think of it this way: If excessive guilt has stopped you from asking for help, it ultimately increases the burden on others, as things may get even worse for everyone without their help.

Feeling Overwhelmed

Feelings associated with being overwhelmed often accompany prolonged illness, especially illness that not only trashes your body, but starts to wear on your mind. Feeling overwhelmed is possibly one of the scariest states to be in, especially when it accompanies the most basic life tasks, everything from everyday grooming to doing the simplest business task. How can you know what help you need when you're physically and mentally exhausted? It is, most definitely, harder.

Once you get caught in overwhelm, it is hard to get out of it. In Step 5, "Slow Down, Don't Move too Fast," I'll go into more detail about how to keep out of this state. For now, the best thing you can do, once you realize that you are feeling overwhelmed, is to take a break. Do something else and take the time to figure out what, exactly, has become too much to handle. If you are having a difficult time thinking it through on your own, ask someone to serve as your sounding board. As I have cautioned before, pick someone who will not give you their advice, at least not right away. Pick someone who listens well and asks good questions. Here is a short list of questions to get you started.

Unraveling Overwhelm

1. Describe what it feels like for you right now.
2. Is there something in particular that is causing confusion?
3. Are there decisions you have to make that you don't know how to make? If so, what help or information do you need?

"COMING OUT"—WHO DO YOU TELL?

When you are ready to tell others what is going on with you, you may still hesitate. At a time when there is endless public chatter about one's personal life, revelation is a more complex question than before. Facebook and Twitter are open forums for sharing, even if with only a few hundred "friends." Some people seem to hold nothing back; others are more guarded, tailoring their public image with caution. In the past, our communities centered around work, family, friends, religion, and a hobby or professional network or two. It was easier to keep things quiet and close to the chest. Even celebrities were afforded more privacy if they liked.

I understand the concerns about privacy and judgment. My personal approach has been to keep my health concerns to myself unless it becomes relevant to others—or unavoidable. When still in the workforce, I did not tell new employers about my health history unless—or until—my symptoms became too much and prevented me from doing my job. As a business owner, even though I don't launch into conversation with clients about my health history, I also don't hide it from them if it becomes relevant to our work together. Years ago, I was so ill that I had to work from bed, which was how the inspiration for the title of this book was born. I certainly didn't announce my work location (under the covers and propped up against pillows) when running marketing "teleclasses" (seminars conducted using telephone conference lines). That would not have been appropriate and served no purpose. However, if it had impacted my ability to lead the class, or was

93

relevant to the participants' growth and development, that would have been another matter.

I have been privy to conversations with people who usually keep illness and pain hidden from the world. Some talk to me in whispered tones, even when no one is around. Because they are vigilantly protective of their reputation, I wonder if they are thwarting their own healing. How can it be good for you to keep something suppressed and hidden that is a real part of your life? How can it help your healing process if you hide a significant aspect of your life circumstances from people who could offer support and understanding? In recent years, various groups of people who had previously kept an essential part of their nature hidden have begun to speak out. Even in the face of some backlash, most say that it was more damaging to hide, and a relief to tell the truth.

I repeat, I am not suggesting that you shout it to the hills and to all who will listen. You are right to be cautious and discerning. When I set out to write *Women, Work, and Autoimmune Disease* with Rosalind, my symptoms had just gone into remission and I was feeling better, more confident, and stronger than I had in years. Even though I had never self-identified as a chronically sick person, I was somewhat concerned that if I were to dive into the topic of the book and talk openly about my illness history, that two things could happen: One, I would somehow be admitting defeat to Crohn's Disease, and, two, that public disclosure of my illness might cause me problems down the line. I don't recall how I reconciled these two concerns, but I do know I decided they were more likely fears than they were foregone conclusions.

The following are the most common reasons given for wanting to keep illness hidden. How many of these describe you?

- Fear of becoming overly-identified with your illness (externally and internally)
- Belief that talking about it will keep your illness locked in place

- Belief that admitting to ill health is a sign of weakness
- A strong sense of self-preservation associated with reactions from overly concerned clients, colleagues, relatives, or friends
- Not wanting to add burden to people you care about
- Fear that once people know they'll think differently about you
- Concerns about loss of business or client loyalty (or losing your job if you're employed)

One business owner I interviewed told me that making the decision about whom to tell and what to tell them were among the most difficult questions to answer. Where do you draw the line? If you have any celebrity at all (i.e., if a lot of people know you in and around your profession or you have a large fan base), to what degree does anyone need to know? Where do your right to privacy end and your obligation to your "fans" begin? Less than a handful of her clients knew what was going on with her. Her business team knew—they had to—and most of her friends did, too. Beyond that, the general public knew nothing.

When I asked about the factors that shaped her decisions about public disclosure, she said that as a business leader with a widespread fan base, she needed to set a strong boundary around her personal space. She understood that people cared about her and that there would be an outpouring of concern. At a time when she was seeking minimal engagement with email and other means of communication, she did not want to add the burden of feeling obligated to reply to notes and messages. In addition, she admitted that she was somewhat concerned about the potential financial impact on her business if people thought she was incapacitated.

Human resource consultant and former vocational rehabilitation counselor, Karen Vandermaas Walsh, owner of KVW HR Solutions, LLC, concurs with the conclusions of this owner. "If clients find out [you are ill] there can be questions about the longevity or the ability of the company to supply services or products. Furthermore, you don't want to scare off good employees, or to be in a position where you can't provide for your employees.…As you take on the role of business owner, you're 'the deal.' You might have administrative assistants and individual contributors and managers, but if you can't do your work the business can be gone, quickly." Walsh elaborated further, "If you want your employees to step up, transparency is important. And, yet, you don't want to lose key people. Some people might foresee a negative impact on the business [and look for employment elsewhere], yet it's a risk you are likely [going] to have to take."

Disclosure Issues for Employees

There are certain protections afforded to you as an employee in that you cannot be let go without cause. Illness presents an interesting situation, though. If it prevents you from doing the job you were hired to do, your employer may have the right to demote you, let you go, or put you in another position. As you know from reading the Prologue, the first two happened to me.

The Americans with Disabilities Act of 1990 (ADA) "makes it unlawful to discriminate in employment against a qualified individual with a disability. The ADA also outlaws discrimination against individuals with disabilities in State and local government services, public accommodations, transportation and telecommunications."[2]

Protections Stipulated in the Americans with Disabilities Act of 1990

The protection offered by the ADA is not without limitations. The following offers greater clarity about the limits of its protection:

"If you have a disability and are qualified to do a job, the ADA protects you from job discrimination on the basis of your disability. Under the ADA, you have a disability if you have a physical or mental impairment that substantially limits a major life activity. The ADA

(continued)

also protects you if you have a history of such a disability, or if an employer believes that you have such a disability, even if you don't.

"To be protected under the ADA, you must have, have a record of, or be regarded as having a substantial, as opposed to a minor, impairment. A substantial impairment is one that significantly limits or restricts a major life activity such as hearing, seeing, speaking, walking, breathing, performing manual tasks, caring for oneself, learning, or working.

"If you have a disability, you must also be qualified to perform the essential functions or duties of a job, with or without reasonable accommodation, in order to be protected from job discrimination by the ADA. This means two things. First, you must satisfy the employer's requirements for the job, such as education, employment experience, skills, or licenses. Second, you must be able to perform the essential functions of the job with or without reasonable accommodation. Essential functions are the fundamental job duties that you must be able to perform on your own or with the help of a reasonable accommodation. An employer cannot refuse to hire you because your disability prevents you from performing duties that are not essential to the job."

The last paragraph holds the key to understanding your rights—"you must be qualified to perform the essential functions or duties of a job." The term, "reasonable accommodation" holds the potential for the greatest area of misinterpretation. We have to be realistic. Companies are run by human beings. Walsh says that, when all is said and done, successful negotiation of adjustments to your schedule and/or workload depend on the people involved, and effective communication. "The employer has to want to work with the employee, and the employee has to really want to work with the employer. Communicating needs and expectations, from a realistic perspective, is critical." Walsh went on to say, "It's much easier if the employee opens the conversation first, before another employee or the manager raises the red flag. There is no legislation that covers this, but when you look at the relationships you have at work, and your employment situation if you want it to continue [working], then it's in your best interest to [initiate] the conversation."

I agree with Walsh. In the two instances where I was either demoted or let go, I recognize my role in the outcomes, in that I failed to inform my employers of my diminishing capacity to perform the essential duties of my job earlier than I could have. Once I understood my limitations—that's the tricky part—I might have been able to minimize the damage and change the outcome if I had been proactive and discussed my illness with either employer earlier on. Yes, hindsight is 20/20. What's more, I still believe everything happened as it should. Life does tend to work itself out, even in the wake of some of the most seemingly undesirable circumstances.

If you do decide that it will be in your best interest to tell someone at work about your situation, depending on the size of the company, you may have one more decision to make, who should you tell? Regarding this decision, Walsh said you have to determine, "Is it best to go to the first line manager (based on the existing relationship) or the [Human Resources] Manager, or even the executive? It's all a matter of where the strongest relationship exists, [and] where the employee can find the best advocate. Because, while discrimination is prohibited by law… the need for flexibility while focusing on abilities—[and] not on 'performance issues'—is required for the successful navigation of this situation."[3]

Americans with Disabilities Act Amendments Act of 2008 (ADAAA)

In 2008, the ADA was amended to include "major bodily functions" (e.g., "functions of the immune system, normal cell growth, digestive, bowel, bladder, neurological, brain, respiratory, circulatory, endocrine, and reproductive functions.")[4] The ADAAA has also extended coverage to employees who have a present or past/history of a disability and also those who are perceived to have a disability or those who associate with an individual with a disability.

(continued)

Employer Size Limits Application of ADAAA

"The ADAAA did not change the basic legal requirement that employers must not discriminate against individuals with disabilities who are qualified for a job, with or without reasonable accommodation."[5] However, there are limits to the application of the ADAAA, in that it applies to companies with 15 or more employees. Companies with less than 15 employees are not required to comply with the regulations, although "State or local laws, however, may apply to smaller employers."[6]

Who Needs to Know?

As with many things in life, there is no singular answer that covers all situations. The following questions will help you develop a list of people or groups that you would like to tell, need to know, and/or can actually be helpful to you in the rebuilding process. Use the questions that follow as a brainstorming tool, for now. Just because someone shows up on your list, doesn't mean you have to tell them.

■ Who will be directly impacted by your illness or injury?
  • Family members
  • Colleagues, clients, or partners
  • Friends
  • Leaders and/or members of organizations to which you belong
■ Who will be concerned if you suddenly "disappear" from your usual activities?
■ What projects will be impacted if you can't perform as you normally do?
  • Direct client work
  • Marketing activities such as newsletters, posts, blogs, etc.
  • Committee or team projects
  • Managing or training others
  • Promises you've made about future projects

■ Who can offer specific support that will help you keep the business afloat?
- Partners
- Family members
- Assistants
- Friends
- Organizations

Don't do anything with this list yet. Wait until you answer the next set of questions before taking any action.

What Do You Say?

Once you've decided who needs to know, either because they will support you in your recovery process or because they will be impacted, you will feel more comfortable if you know what you want to tell people when the time comes. You'll want to modify your approach, depending on whom you're talking to and the medium you're using to communicate. You'll not be able to control all conversations, but you can prepare yourself in order to minimize your anxiety and then compose the message when the time comes.

Use the following questions to help you formulate your communications about your situation:

■ What is the nature of your illness or injury?
- How would you describe what you're dealing with in the simplest terms possible?
- Does it make sense to tell people what the diagnosis is, or do you prefer to speak in more general terms? If you prefer to speak in more general terms, can you describe your situation in ten or fewer words?
■ How does your illness or injury impact you at this moment in time?
- Does it limit your time available to work?
- Does it—or do the medical procedures and medications—impair your mental functioning?
- Can you predict your energy and mood swings or do they vary from day-to-day?

- Are you limited socially?
- Is this a finite situation, or is the timeline for recovery open-ended?

■ How do you want people to interact with you?
  - Do you want to receive help only when you ask for it?
  - Do you want the people you tell to reach out to you if some time has passed and they've not heard from you? If so, how long should they wait?
  - If you want them to treat you as they always have, how can you assure them that this is best and is really okay?
  - Are you comfortable if the people you tell share the information with common acquaintances, or do you want to have full authority over who knows and when?

■ What other requests or guidelines do you want to share with the people you tell?

■ How do your responses to the above questions differ depending on your "audience?"
  - Family and friends closest to you
  - Family and friends who might find out, but are not among people you rely on or see on a regular basis.
  - Business team
  - Clients and customers
  - Business colleagues
  - Social media friends and acquaintances

■ Does it make sense to release information to the general public? If yes, do you need help crafting the message and deciding on the best time? Who should you tell before this information is made public?

Prioritize Your Disclosure List

After answering the questions above, organize the people you identified in your brainstorming list under "Who Needs to Know?" into the following groups:

- Must know
- Would like to know (or you would like them to know)
- Only if they ask
- Never needs to know

TIMING IS EVERYTHING—WHEN DO YOU TELL?

The timing will vary and depend largely on your own acceptance and understanding of your situation. As many people do, you may be able to hide your condition for quite a long time or forever. Some people never need to know. You have the right to make those decisions.

You don't have to tell everyone at once. You can pace yourself and start with the inner-most circle first. You can start with the people who must know—and you would like to know—and allow the rest to unfold over time. If it supports your efforts, develop a communication plan. I always like to start with the easiest people first, signified by my sense that they will hear me without overreacting, ask intelligent questions, and offer the kind of support I need. If there are people who need to know, but whom you would prefer never to tell, you can ask someone you trust to help you prepare what you'll say to these people.

WHAT HELP DO YOU NEED?

Once you decide whom you will tell, and what you will say, it will be easier to think about what assistance you need and from whom. Obviously, some people—such as your new housekeeper or plumber—may never need to know why you need their help. Use the following questions to assess your needs:

Everyday Living

- What are the everyday tasks that are essential to your welfare and make you feel good? *Examples:* brushing your teeth (I know, simple), showering, cooking, etc.
- What are the everyday tasks that feel good to do but are less than essential? *Examples:* getting dressed, making your bed, cleaning dishes, etc.

■ What are the everyday tasks that are essential but are difficult to execute? *Examples:* anything you put on the two lists above that are not easy at this moment in time.

Everyday Business

■ Which everyday business tasks are most important, and are easy and fun to do? *Examples:* customer interactions, email communication, order fulfillment, etc.
■ Which everyday business tasks are essential, but feel overwhelming at the moment? *Examples:* can be the same as the list above, depending on what is fun and how you feel.
■ What everyday business tasks can be put off until you're feeling more energetic? *Examples:* new projects of any kind, some marketing activities, new purchases, etc.

The examples I've given for everyday business tasks may be very different than your lists. They will vary greatly depending on your business or job, and the ways in which your illness or injury limits you. If your replies to the previous questions have not yet clarified your needs, ask a trusted business confidante (coach, partner, or colleague) or friend or family member to help you finalize your lists.

Sometimes, no matter what you do, the answers are not immediately clear. If you push too hard, it may increase your sense of overwhelm and anxiety. When the answer is not immediate, you may only need to let go and let things be. Yes, sometimes the best course of action is no action. With a day or two more, without pushing for a resolution, clarity often comes and your true priorities will become clear.

BRING IT HOME—WHO DO YOU ASK TO HELP WITH WHAT?

You've met Peggy in earlier chapters. Learning to allow, receive, and ask for help were among the greatest "gifts" of her illness experience. She told me that when she started her chemotherapy treatments she thought she would go to them by herself. Even though this might seem like a ridiculous notion to most of us, Peggy has always been more at ease offering help than asking for it.

But, one day, when visiting with her adult son, she found herself asking if he would like to go with her to her treatment, to which he readily replied, "Yes, I would like to do that. I didn't think you'd ask." Peggy had assumed that if her son wanted to go with her he would volunteer that information and offer to go. Her son had assumed that if she wanted him with her she would ask. We have a case where two people wanted the same thing, but in the silence of no communication, neither would have gotten what they really wanted. If that "wall of assumption" had persisted, a sense of loneliness and distance might have filled the air between them, which might have turned into regret and, possibly, resentment.

Who knows what quiet nudge prompted Peggy to ask her son if he would like to go with her? I'm just glad she paid attention and opened her mouth. I heard the joy in her voice when she told me he went to every treatment thereafter. It's easy to imagine the peaceful communion between them during this difficult time.

Peggy said in conclusion, "Yes, you're fine [in the big picture sense of all-is-well] but it's okay to ask for help. If you don't, you don't allow the other person the joy of giving when they can." On the other side of the equation, she says to those who would like to help but don't know how, don't wait. "Ask, don't assume." I hope that Peggy will remember this as she continues to regain her strength. That's the real trick.

Just as all employees and owners are not created equally, the same goes for caretakers. Some people are very good with practical, tactical tasks, and others are better at providing emotional support. Just as an owner needs to hire people with the right skills, as the manager of your health and well-being, you can be selective about whom you ask for help, too.

Table 4.1 shows you how you can organize your list of tasks and projects, match them with people who could help, and remind yourself of their relative priority. I recommend that you create a similar table in your journal or in a Word document on your computer, one for business, and one for personal tasks and projects. I've inserted examples to jumpstart your thinking. In answer to

TABLE 4.1
Who Can I Ask for Help?

Tasks You Need Help With	How Frequently?	Who May Be Able to Help?	How Important Is It? (High, Medium, Low)
Business Tasks			
Review and prioritize email	30 minutes a day	Virtual assistant, college student	Medium
Edit and distribute blog posts and articles	2 hours a week	Virtual assistant, intern, marketing manager	High
Pay bills and invoice customers	2 times a month	Spouse, bookkeeper, virtual assistant	High
Manage social media presence	3 times a week	Virtual assistant, social media manager, techie teenage daughter	Low
Personal Tasks			
Laundry	3 hours a week	Spouse, son	High
Grocery shopping	2 hours a week	Online grocer, neighbor, spouse	High
Clean the gutter of leaves	2 times a year	Lawn care specialist, daughter, spouse	Medium
Drive to medical appointments	2–3 times a month	Spouse, neighbor, parent	High

the question, "How important is it?" the priority rating is yours to make. For example, if, in your life, laundry is a low priority, note it as such. The examples are just that, examples.

APPROACH MATTERS—COMMUNICATION AND RESPECT

If you make requests for help in a straightforward manner, without expectations and without apology, you'll probably feel better about asking and get a better response, too. Here are a few things to keep in mind when you ask for help.

- Does the person you are asking for help have the ability (skills and time) to carry out your request?
- Is it something you need help with on a strict schedule or is it something that can be scheduled at the person's convenience?
- Does the person you're asking need something you have the capacity to offer in return?
- Do you need to—and can you—pay for this service? If so, what is your budget?
- Can you find someone to do it for free? If so, what are the potential problems?

Charles, a personal financial advisor and business owner in the San Francisco area, has a good partnership with his wife, who was diagnosed with multiple sclerosis in 1995. I was impressed by the manner in which he and his wife seem to have negotiated the balance of give and take in their relationship. She is able to do quite a bit on her own, but he offers support in the evening hours when she is physically weaker, and during the morning shower routine, which requires difficult position transfers, even when two caregivers are assisting. Charles made it clear that, while he gives care, he receives it in return. He offers her much-needed physical support and he relies on his wife's superior memory and organizational skills to move their joint tasks to completion. Furthermore, he says that it is her energetic personality and drive, even in the face of an energy-sapping disease, that have been instrumental in developing a path through life that has more positives than would otherwise be possible.

They were fortunate (and smart), as they had purchased Long-Term Care insurance before she became ill. The benefits have enabled them to utilize the services of home health care aides on a regular basis, making life easier for both of them. Charles explained:

> The aides have 11 hours/week of regularly scheduled visits, and I am usually home when they are working with my wife...their presence frees me up from hands-on care-giving to do other tasks in the home or yard. When I have to be away for business or pleasure, we schedule additional hours for the aides, who then cover both direct care-giving and household tasks that I am unable to do.

They were equally fortunate in that Charles made the decision early in his business to hire and groom three other financial advisors to help him serve clients and run the business. He didn't do this in anticipation of what was to come, but because he wanted to be part of a team instead of a solo business owner. Coincidentally, by the time his wife started needing more care he was able to adjust his working hours accordingly.

These are the two practical elements that make it possible for Charles to be of assistance to his wife when she needs it. It is Charles' ability to continue to carve out time for his needs and personal interests that impressed me most. He goes to the gym a couple of times a week, something that makes him feel good and also helps maintain his strength, which he needs to help his wife move from one location to the next. He's been practicing yoga for two years and was able to take advantage of a weekend retreat. In order to do this, he and his wife took the necessary steps to get someone to come into their home for a couple of days, through the long-term care company. Again, we see a strong partnership. She figures out when the extra help will be needed and drafts the requests. He proofs the requests and sends them out.

Charles enjoys travel photography, too, and recently traveled to the Galapagos Islands. For these longer trips, they add family members and friends to the mix of caregivers so that his wife is able to spend some of that time with her closest circle of family and friends. He mentioned his gratitude that he and his wife did their fair share of traveling in earlier years, before she became ill. They do still travel together, but more often than not they take shorter trips in their van to make it easier for both of them.

As a primary caregiver, Charles has not suppressed his personal needs and interests, turning himself into a sacrificial lamb—quite the opposite. His wife has a great deal to contribute to this equation, too. She not only accepts his help, she understands and actively supports his pursuit of the recreational activities that help keep him happy, refreshed, and renewed. In order to do this she has had to allow other people into her home, people she may not feel as comfortable with as she does with Charles. Clearly, he and his wife have adapted to their situation so they both get their needs met.

With more clarity about the kind of help you need, and armed with insight about who to tell and what you want to tell them, you'll be in a stronger position to rebuild your business—and your life—in a way that is more sustainable and satisfying than it was before you became ill. No one I spoke with said that they did it alone or that their orientation to their priorities did not change.

5 Things to Remember, Try, and Discard

5 Things to Remember

1. Asking for help is smart.
2. Accepting help is a gift that you allow another person to give you.
3. You have a right to get the help you need.
4. You don't have to tell everyone, but...
5. Some people can be trusted with your truth.

5 Things to Try

1. Eliminate one task or project that is non-essential.
2. Tell someone, who doesn't yet know, what your life is like right now. Include a gory detail or two.
3. Choose two business tasks or projects to outsource to someone else.
4. Choose two home-based tasks or projects that you'll ask someone to help you with.
5. Thank someone who has been helping already. Tell them what it means to you.

5 Things to Discard

1. Guilt
2. Shame
3. Lone wolf behavior
4. Stoicism
5. The notion that to be worthy is to always be "on"

Step 5:
Slow Down, Don't Move Too Fast

*Deep healing cannot be forced...but must be allowed to take place
at its own pace.*
—David Nortman, Homeopathic Practitioner

Throughout this book, and through each of the four previous steps,
I've encouraged you to slow down and modulate your return to
"normal life." You may have seen the light, yourself, thinking and
feeling the wisdom of such an approach. I also know, from my years
studying human behavior (first in college, then through a variety of
human development training programs, and finally, through working directly with determined entrepreneurs), that there is a gap
between knowing what is healthy and actually taking the actions to
change behavior that will assist with healing. Habitual patterns of
thinking, external pressures to conform, and fear of potential consequences, all work together to challenge you.

I blame the fax machine. Even before email became the
standard for correspondence in business, the use of fax machines
started to chip away at our tolerance for waiting. Before, we had to

wait for at least a day—if not two or three—to receive an important document, but with arrival of the fax, we had only to wait a few minutes. Suddenly, we could transmit information across the globe—or at least across the country—in a matter of seconds or minutes. Rather than reducing our level of stress, as intended, modern conveniences have increased it. They have created an ever-increasing performance gap. We are still people and we operate at people speed, not transmission speed, but we have forgotten that.

When I asked the people I interviewed what they'd want to see in a book like this, most said they were aware of their need to change their approach. Some were in the process of making significant changes, and quite successfully. Others were having a harder time. Either way, most wished that they'd had some guidance about how to balance their drive to get back to work with their wish to live a more consciously healthy life. The guidance and experiences shared in Step 5 will help you uncover what will work for you in your life.

MIND AND HEART ARE RARING TO GO, BODY NOT AS MUCH

> The biggest frustration has been getting my body and mind to coordinate with each other. My mind thinks my body can do more than it knows it can. I think I have more energy than I do. I plan things and I make my to-do list and my body says, "Are you out of your mind?" That's the thing, my energy is slow to come back and I try to push it. Your body won't let you push it; your body will only allow you so much.

Peggy's experience reflected that of many others I interviewed for this book, and reflects my experience, too. There will be a turning point in your health crises where, for the first time in weeks or months, you get a glimmer of wellness. You notice that your energy has increased and you feel a little stronger and more optimistic. After months—or years—of living in the shadow of continuous pain and lack of energy, you feel ready to take on the world. But, you soon realize you're not ready, at least not all at once. Instead, you enter into a frustrating and confusing battle between your mind, your heart, and your body.

Peggy hit the nail on the head when she explained, "The mind doesn't pay attention to anybody else. Your mind says 'I'm important, I'm important.' But your body says, 'You've got to listen to me!' Mind says, 'No, I don't, I can do anything I can put my mind to.' But, when you put your mind to it, your body had better be ready to go with you."

We are shaped by the environment we work in, an environment where speed and determination dominate. We have been acculturated to a belief that you "get back on that horse" as soon as you can. "Don't let the grass grow under your feet." Furthermore, if you have been confined to your home for long stretches of time, your spirit responds like the prisoner who is finally released back into the world. It makes sense that you feel exhilarated upon the first glimmers of release from your unwanted confinement; the rush to "get back to work" is reasonable. When you add a significant loss in revenue to the mix, you've certainly got the ingredients for a strong dose of internal pressure. Despite these feelings, powering through the workday isn't viable anymore. Your body is your master now, and it will be hard to ignore this fact without paying the price.

Professional writer Kristina Anderson was determined—and had the means—to keep her business afloat during the year in which she underwent chemotherapy treatments following a double mastectomy. Through the use of sub-contractors, she was able to divvy up the workload during the most difficult months. As you'll read, it wasn't easy for her to stay still at the first sign of "release" from the worst of the side effects.

My diagnosis was in mid-March of 2008 and I finished treatment in June of 2009. I went back to work—what I would say is full time—but I still struggled. I definitely was fatigued. I was coming off the Herceptin…it targets the *HER2* genes [which promotes cancer growth] in your body, including…the lining of your heart. So I had heart issues, and that affected my breathing. There was a heavy feeling in my chest, so I worked but I had a hard time.

I interviewed Kristina in early 2012, two-plus years after her last treatment. She and I talked just a couple of weeks after an intense period of work. She went on to say:

I just came off of two intense months [of work]. In January and February I put in a huge number of hours on several projects, and on one in particular. That project ended on February 1st, and I was able to keep up. I was juicing twice a day, I made sure I was walking my dog, four miles an hour for an hour every day. No matter what, I still walked. I told my clients, "I'm taking a break. I really need to get away from the office, but I'll be back in an hour or so." I did great. I was still high energy until a few days afterwards.

Almost 2 weeks ago tomorrow, I crashed. I haven't gotten back to "normal" yet. I'm taking afternoon naps again. But, I made sure that my health was the priority. I could work 12 hour days. I got up at 5 and went to bed at midnight. I was able to keep up.

When listening to Kristina talk about her experience, I was impressed by the drive that propelled her towards working long hours and struck by the significance of her body-crash afterwards. It reminded me, once again, of the power of the mind to override the body to the point of exhaustion.

At this point in my life, modulating my energy outflow is second nature to me—I don't think about it anymore, I just do it. When I notice my energy ebb, I stop what I am doing even if I'm not "done" for the day. Minimally, I take a break or change my location. If my energy returns, I continue on. If it doesn't, I don't. That wasn't always the case. I had to learn to read the signs and to make self-care a higher priority.

I already told you about the absurd level of responsibility I took on when I first became ill. Understandably, I was in complete denial of my situation. In late 1995, shortly after being let go following the 10-day disability leave I mentioned in the Prologue, I got a new job as an executive assistant and marketing coordinator for a new national women's business organization. I started as a part-time employee and worked my way up to full-time within a couple of months. During this period, my symptoms remained in remission. Since the president and I were the two sole employees, there was a lot of work to do and, though I was able to work from home at times, I also put in excessively long hours on several occasions, including a few overnights.

I was not aware of how many overtime hours I'd accumulated until we lost our major source of funding in 1997 and I was laid off. The organization was required to pay me for seven solid weeks of overtime (accumulated in 1997) before letting me go. Seven weeks at 40 hours a week equates to 280 hours! Fortunately, I did not become ill that year, but I look back with wonder at the level of dedication and drive we both exhibited. That was only 4 years into my roller coaster ride with Crohn's. I was feeling quite hopeful about my prognosis, and thought I had good reason to.

The next year, 1998, was a difficult year, health wise. It didn't take me long to find another position, this time as an assistant recruiter working directly with the owner of a one-man placement service company. While I was going about the business of working and living my life, my body developed a fistula, a sign of aggressive Crohn's Disease, and I developed the two "spontaneous" infections in my right foot that I mentioned in Step 3. It would be irresponsible of me to draw a direct connection between all that overtime in 1997 and the unpleasant symptoms that showed up the next year. But, clearly, there was some kind of imbalance continuing to run in the background. I think it fair to say that I had not yet learned to put my health and personal priorities ahead of the drive to appear reliable and trustworthy. I was still learning.

STRESS AND ILLNESS RECOVERY

*Stress never comes directly from your circumstances. It comes from
your thoughts about your circumstances.*
—ANDREW BERNSTEIN, *THE MYTH OF STRESS*

The conditions for your illness were not ignited in a vacuum. While
you were pursuing your goals, your body was absorbing the impact
of all manners of stress: emotional, psychic, mental, and environmental. When chronic stress becomes normal you stop perceiving
it, but that doesn't mean it's not there. Stress—environmental, psychological, or physical—may not have caused your illness, but you
can be sure it either contributed to its eruption or aggravates your
symptoms today.

The Biochemistry Behind Stress—The Role of Adrenaline

Good old adrenaline. Having served us well for centuries on end,
when physical survival was an everyday event, it has become a
leading culprit in many physical ailments in our less physically
demanding lives. Adrenaline gives you that push you feel when
you are required—or require yourself—to engage in activities
that pump you up or push you beyond your limits. It doesn't
take much of a push for adrenaline to kick in. Any time you are
surprised or spurred into activity, adrenaline is pumped into
your body.

Adrenaline, one of two hormones produced in response to
physical or psychological stress, plays a role in your ability to heal
(or not heal). As you'll see, your ability to modulate your levels
of stress will help keep this hormone in check. You'll also get a
glimpse into the degree of rigor required to do so. If you insist on
returning to work before you're physically ready, you may be able
to for a short period of time—adrenaline will help—but you will
eventually find yourself back in bed.

Adrenaline doesn't cause stress. It is a chemical produced by your adrenal glands and released into your body in response to a perceived threat, real or otherwise. The cue to initiate its release starts with the hypothalamus, a tiny pearl-sized receptor in your brain. Your *perception* of potentially dangerous situations ignites the response to release this hormone. Associated with the famous "fight or flight" response, adrenaline gives you much-needed boosts of energy and strength in true emergencies. It is a useful hormone in that it enables you to escape danger more quickly and with greater strength and speed than your body would otherwise be able to do.

In the past, when humans lived in closer proximity to the animal kingdom, the sudden flood of adrenaline into the bloodstream at the sight or sound of external threats was critical to survival. It got the muscles of our ancestors moving quickly in order to get out of harm's way, or to kill the threatening presence. In other words, the adrenaline response was perfectly designed to protect you from immediate harm.

It takes a conscious effort to shut the "imminent danger" thought process off. In *Steering by Starlight*, Martha Beck reminds us that "a wild reptile may react to predators by running away in a panic, but once the predators are gone, the reptile doesn't sit around brooding about the dreadfulness of the experience. Its fight or flight reactions abate quickly, allowing its body and brain to rest until the next emergency requires quick action." A lizard would never brood about the "dreadfulness of the experience." But we brood, don't we?

The *perceived* threats we live with today don't last for just a few minutes. For most of us living in the developed world, stress levels are chronically high. As safe as we are from the eat-or-be-eaten predators of our ancestors, we think, act, and respond as if the bear is standing on the other side of the door. Influenced by "the news," and extraordinary pressure to succeed and get ahead and get things done, our stress responses have gone into overdrive.

117

To be fair, stress is neither inherently positive nor inherently negative. However, the emotions associated with the source of stress can be either, depending on your orientation. For example, the increased heart-rate and sweaty palms that you feel in anticipation of an upcoming special event can be interpreted as either fear or excitement. New love, new friendship, and the thrill of the sale, all have the potential to increase the release of adrenaline into your blood stream. The adrenaline response is not usually threatening to your health in short spurts when followed by long periods of rest.

Continuous production of adrenaline with little rest between episodes, however, leads to a variety of health issues. In his book, *The Hidden Link Between Adrenaline and Stress*, Dr. Archibald Hart tells us that "Bursts of adrenaline give us a buzz or feeling of excitement. But when you don't get a chance to unwind from stress, when the battering of adrenaline and other stress hormones continues without a break, the body goes into overdrive. The result is a drain on your body's vital systems."[1]

Cortisol, the Other Stress-Response Hormone

In addition to adrenaline, your adrenal glands also produce the hormone cortisol, an essential anti-inflammatory hormone. "Cortisol functions to reduce inflammation in the body, which is good, but over time, these efforts to reduce inflammation also suppress the immune system. Chronic inflammation, caused by lifestyle factors such as poor diet and stress, helps to keep cortisol levels soaring, wreaking havoc on the immune system."[2] Inflammatory conditions are strongly correlated with a wide range of illnesses, everything from persistent laryngitis to any one of the 63 autoimmune illnesses. If you have ever been given steroids (for example, prednisone or prednisolone) to treat the symptoms associated with your illness, you are likely to have experienced the miraculous reversal of your symptoms. According to Dr. James L. Wilson, "these drugs imitate the anti-inflammatory effects of cortisol."[3]

Cortisol is involved in several essential body functions, as follows: glucose metabolism, regulation of blood pressure, insulin release, immune function, and inflammatory response. Cortisol helps in true emergencies by flooding the body with glucose, supplying an immediate energy source to large muscles. In order to keep your cortisol levels functioning in the normal range, a return to a resting state after the fight-or-flight response is needed.

I consulted former nurse turned lifestyle and wellness coach, Dina Markind, to ask about the role cortisol plays in the stress and health equation. Dina said, "If your body is chronically exposed to [too much] cortisol, you're going to have similar effects as long-term exposure to steroids: muscle atrophy, increased gastro-intestinal distress, high blood sugar, and an increased risk of brittle bones." In addition, chronic over-production of cortisol, instead of reducing inflammation, increases inflammatory conditions in the body and puts fat squarely over your vital organs, around your heart and on your belly.

How Does Adrenaline Fool Us?

Continuous adrenaline production is a symptom of everyday busyness and is released into your body when you get into those crunchy deadline situations. It creates a false sense of energy after your normal reserves have been depleted. It's the chemical that has you say, "I do my best work under pressure" or "one more hour won't hurt me."

Adrenaline is addictive. When the pressures associated with an excessive schedule disappear, the sudden reduction in adrenaline leaves you feeling lethargic. Without a steady flow of adrenaline, some people actually become bored. Mistaking boredom for depression or lack of motivation, adrenaline addicts are prone to create "emergencies" just to feel better again.

Unfortunately, we unknowingly create adrenaline-pumping emergencies every time our thoughts project danger where there is none. Below are a few examples of the kinds of thoughts that you may have, consciously or not, that would ignite an emergency-response where there is none. The first, or some version of it, is especially common.

- "I'm really busy right now, but it's better than the alternative."
- "I can't rest now; I have a deadline to meet."
- "If I don't get back to work now I'll end up on the street."

If you never stop to ask yourself, "Am I OK today, at this very moment?" you are likely to project danger into an unknown future, often unnecessarily.

How Do You Know When to Yield to Your Body and When to Push Through?

It can take a frustratingly long time for a body to heal after a significant health setback. The mind, heart, and spirit long for a return to normal. As Dr. JoAnn LeMaistre wrote in an online adaptation of her book, *After the Diagnosis*, "It is not necessary to like or to resign yourself to the compromises you need to make to get on with living. It is only necessary to acknowledge that changes in life style and skills have to be made. Acknowledging that your skills are different from your pre-illness days is not the same as 'adjusting' to illness. There is no surrender involved, only growth—the creation of new options through new means."[4]

Your stress monsters will be different than mine. Your body responses to stress will be different, too. The trick, of course, is to learn how to read the signs, to know when it is okay to push a little further and when it is best to slow down or stop working all together. In the process of learning what works for you, you will not only need to modulate your physical energy, you will also need to adjust your mental and emotional thermostat to align with your updated reality. Depending on the nature of your illness or injury, you may be required to remain continuously vigilant in order to maintain overall wellness. My aim is to help you understand the process by asking questions and sharing experiences that will support you as you experiment with and adjust to these changes.

HEALING GUIDANCE FROM A RUBBER BAND

Picture a rubber band for a moment. With very little tension, it sits there "doing nothing," lying on your desk somewhat formless and lifeless. At first glance, you might think it's not very useful in this state. However, I'd like to think that the rubber band at rest could be equated to the moments in our lives when we are quiet and calm, either in a meditative state or enjoying a good night's sleep.

Put that rubber band to work and it immediately starts to stretch. What happens when you wrap it around a rolled up piece of paper? If it's the right size and width and you wrap it just the right number of times, it becomes an effective tool for keeping that paper rolled up for years on end, or at least until the rubber wears out and looses elasticity. (You know, like aging.)

Now think about the same rubber band when it's stretched out further than is optimal. Imagine pulling it wide with your fingers or wrapping it around the same rolled up piece of paper one too many times. What is likely to happen, if not right away, eventually? It wears out or it breaks.

Now, replace the rubber band with you, giving it a brain with the ability to measure, assess, and modulate. You, like the rubber band, are feeling just the "right" level of tension as you go about your work. In an optimal state of stress or tension:

- You are able to work for a reasonable length of time.
- You are patient and trusting, feeling no pressure to rush or force the outcomes.

- When you reach your limit you stop working and do something else.
- You are comfortable with the idea that you are perfectly suited for specific tasks and not as well for others. (A rubber band is not a hammer, after all.)
- If something—or someone—comes along that threatens to disturb the calm, you feel the tension increase but your reactions are brief. You adjust as needed.

Stress and the Rubber Band—Warning, Warning

When you stretch that rubber band—or yourself—beyond its structural capacity, stress and tension increase. Stretch it too much or for too long and the rubber band breaks. What happens to you?

- You feel the strain but you keep pressing on.
- You risk your well-being for the promise of the outcome.
- You might think—consciously or not—that if you stop to rest you'll never get that tension back.
- You increase the chances of making mistakes that will require you go back and fix them later.
- You're likely to chase results, only to find they elude you.

You can't expect to remain motionless any more than you can expect to operate for long periods at maximum capacity. You wouldn't want to. Life is always changing, and you are, too. We grow through stress. However, we don't grow through unrelenting stress. Through different experiences you establish new set points; sometimes they are lower and sometimes they are higher. Well-tuned bodies operate quite well within an optimal level of stress.

Next time you feel tired, remember the rubber band. Perhaps you're only stretched a little too far for longer than you can actually withstand. Pull back a little and feel the tension disappear. Imagine your body (emotional and physical) plumping right back up, relaxed, and functional. Take all the time you need.

Self-Discovery

1. Identify the most prominent fear-based thought, the one that is creating the greatest amount of pressure and stress in your life.
   a. First, give into it completely. What is the very worst thing that could happen? What could you do if it did?
   b. Now, argue for the other side and see if you can't find some evidence that it may, in fact, be an exaggerated thought or entirely untrue in the moment.
2. Identify one thing you can do to eliminate one ounce of busyness from your life. Eliminate it now. Just stop doing it.
3. Educate yourself. Do some research to gain a clearer understanding of the role excess adrenaline plays in reduced health and well-being. Start with these three keywords in your favorite search engine: adrenaline health problems.

THE UN-HURRY MANTRA—BUSINESS SUCCESS IN THE SLOWER LANE

Earlier in the book, in Step 2, I mentioned a woman named Joelle who, after a two-month disability leave, returned to her job only to discover that she'd slowed down considerably. Her posture had changed, she walked at a slower pace and her head was more squarely centered over her body than it had been in years. The difference was significantly palpable to her. She committed to herself that she would not return to her former posture. I would say that Joelle adopted the "Un-Hurry Mantra."

The "Un-Hurry Mantra" will help you return to business in a more mindful way, and at a pace that will increase the likelihood that you will reach a level of productivity that is satisfactory and sustainable. There are few times in life when you're given an opportunity to test your assumptions about the recipe for success. This is one of them. Do you *have* to get back to doing things at the same pace as before you became ill or injured? Must you do things the way you've always done them to enjoy your life and succeed in business? Are the values of your peers, parents, and society your values, or are yours different?

Peggy, the mortgage loan officer, commented on her own change in attitude. "I'm not out every night of the week at meetings. I've learned to say "no" to things that would be better to allow others to take the lead on. I try to get more rest. I still have difficulty sleeping but I still try to get more rest. I try to plan around my energy pockets if you know what I mean."

The "Un-Hurry Mantra" gives you access to asking and answering these questions for yourself. Most of the entrepreneurs I interviewed said that they did learn to slow down, and that doing so was not only okay, but more satisfying. Kelly McClelland, a transition coach, entrepreneur, and missionary, was derailed from his life plan when a heart condition, aggravated by extreme reactive hypoglycemia, required he and his wife discontinue their missionary work in Indonesia and return home to the United States. It took quite a few tests, a few medical experts, and independent research before Kelly was able to grasp the severity of his situation. The turning point came when a particularly straightforward doctor reviewed his medical tests and said,

> If you want a short ministry, keep doing what you're doing. With the state your heart is in, and your predisposition, your body can't take the highs and lows that you're getting. Those sweats that you're having, and the incapacitation afterwards, are warning signals. I'd give you between 6 and 18 months because you're going to die. Your heart is going to give out.

Kelly, taking the prognosis seriously, set out to secure work back at home. Prior to the missionary work he was a corporate head hunter. Knowing the value of a good network, Kelly reached out to his mission community and scheduled fourteen interviews, starting just two weeks after his return home. About halfway through the interview process he was offered a position with Pioneers International. Six months later, he underwent quadruple bypass surgery.

Instead of feeling bitter, Kelly exhibits resilience untainted by resentment. His faith, as well as his life experiences, have buoyed his ability to go with the flow of life events. When I asked him what is different, now that he is on the healing side of these critical events, he replied:

> I see major shifts in the way I approach life. One, I've learned to take deep breaths...When I say deep breaths, I allow myself room—sometimes maybe too much—but I don't push myself as hard. During my recovery time I [rediscovered] things I used to ignore and neglect in my life. With the fast pace of the ministry work we were extremely busy, and on call all the time. I had let go of hobbies and interests, things like reading and having fun.

> I'm a ham operator, and have been since I was 12 years old. I hadn't done it for years and I decided "it's time to go back." I found a real joy in that. I love being outdoors, and I combine that with my hobby. Every morning I take a walk down by the lake. I check out the fish and the snakes and the birds, and I just love it. I didn't do that throughout most of my business and ministry career. That always took a back seat. So, that's a major change and we love it. My wife, I think, is much happier with me, too.

I also talked to a few people who are less convinced that working at a slower, more tempered pace is either ideal or preferable. Among this group is an entrepreneur in his early seventies who was undergoing his second round of chemotherapy treatments after a relatively short period of remission. His is a "work until you drop" approach. (These are his words, not mine.) He is not alone in this. There are plenty of people who ascribe to the idea that, if they only have a short time on this earth, they want to be "used up" when it's their time to go.

I am not telling you that you should not re-engage with enthusiasm. I am inviting you to give yourself a chance to fully recover. It takes time for your body to heal. Mine was a chronic and fluctuating situation for thirteen years. Even when I was able to go about my life at a fairly normal pace, doing fairly normal things, I was still weak. I could feel it even when others couldn't see it.

Like you, I never gave up. I did everything possible to recover my health while I was trying to build my business. In addition to my coaches, mentors, and medical doctors, in 2004 I sought counsel from a medical intuitive named Janet. Janet told me that for every year I'd been sick—12 years at the time—I would need to engage in some kind of deep healing work for one entire month. Translation: I would need to engage in deep healing work for an entire year.

Janet's guidance is based on the healing principles of homeopathic medicine. Rather than suppressing symptoms, homeopathy seeks to treat and heal the underlying source of illness. The one-month-for-every-year rule is not a definitive prescription. Various factors influence the speed of healing, including genetic predisposition, current levels of stress, the initial source of the imbalance, emotional resiliency, and your attitude and beliefs towards life, health, and healing. According to homeopathic and naturopathic doctor, David Norton, "Deep healing…demands the conscious and unconscious participation of the patient, since progress is affected by the degree of readiness to get better, and there are unpredictable stresses in the physical and social environments that can further hinder progress."[5] Just like there is no one-size-fits-all in business, there is no one-size-fits-all in healing.

Janet recommended I try Reiki, but after doing some research I decided I wasn't sufficiently interested in that modality to pursue it. Yet, I felt the wisdom in her counsel, and shortly thereafter I was introduced to another form of energy work, network spinal analysis (NSA).[6] I interviewed the practitioner I was referred to and liked what he told me about NSA as much as I liked his manner and approach. He and I were able to work out a trade and I committed to work with him for a year on a schedule I could manage.

Within three months I noticed a change in my energy. My symptoms had all but disappeared and I felt good. After six months, in June 2005, when my husband and I took a trip to Boston and walked the Freedom Trail, I realized I was stronger than I'd been in years. Previously when he and I took vacations, we could not count on my health. We have had to abort more than one trip, or reduce the level of activity we had planned, because I would either run out of energy or have a full-blown flare up. I had been well at other times, but right there, on that Freedom Trail, I knew with every ounce of my being that the improvement was significant. I did not feel frail. I felt strong. Three months after that, when I had my biannual colonoscopy, my gastroenterologist confirmed what I felt. My symptoms had gone into remission.

Having made the commitment to one year of healing work, I continued as planned. I lived about 20–25 minutes away from the NSA practitioner so it took about 90 minutes of my time for each visit. It would have been easy to convince myself that I didn't need to continue to interrupt my business day with NSA after the gastroenterologist confirmed that my symptoms had gone into remission. But, I didn't stop going. I felt it was the right thing to do, and I was empowered by my decision to put my health first, to remain "unhurried."

BODY BREAKS

As I mentioned earlier, modulating my energy output has become second nature to me. When it comes to this practice, you could say that I am unconsciously competent. None of us start out at this level of mastery. Competence increases in stages:

1. Unconscious and incompetent (in other words, clueless)
2. Conscious and incompetent (now, at least you know you don't know what you're doing)
3. Conscious and competent (you're competent in the new skill or habit but you still have to think about it)
4. The final level of "mastery," unconsciously competent (it's become second nature to you)

If you find yourself mentally rushing to get back to work, scheduling body breaks—moments during the day where you focus on your body and its needs—will help you remain more centered and mindful while you rebuild your business and restore your health. Although a body break can definitely include exercise, it does not inherently have to be exercise. This is because exercise, in the healthy world, tends to mimic the push mentality of today's business world. We don't just have yoga anymore, we have hot yoga. We don't have cycling classes, we have spin cycling (pedaling on a stationary bike as fast as you can for 60 minutes). I am not philosophically averse to intense exercise (or maybe I am), but I worry that our ideas about exercise have become infused with the same "should" mentality as so many other things in life. Furthermore, what is appropriate for a healthy person is not appropriate for someone who has been laid up in bed for a prolonged period of time. Hot yoga, as healthy as it is, can tax a weak body system.

After a prolonged illness, your body is weak. It has been weakened by the chronic nature of the fight to heal. During your illness a significant amount of your biophysical energy was directed towards your body's efforts to repair the damaged system. Any medications you take—or took—have altered your chemistry, and your muscles have either atrophied or morphed in response to pain. If you pay attention, you'll notice that under the renewed sense of wellness you can detect a certain degree of weakness.

What Is the Purpose of a Body Break?

Body breaks are meant to do three things:

1. Rebuild your physical strength so that your recovery is not just fleeting, but sustainable
2. Install new habits so that as you increase your productive capacity, you continue to mind your body
3. Help you tune into what is right in your world, thus reducing the tendency to inject your actions with worry-based responses

Any time you put attention on your body, you gain access to the source of your wisdom and power. Through body breaks, you will be better able to observe the body-patterns that have been locked in place, and you are more likely to find peace in the moment.

Try it now. Just sit still and take a deep breath. Take more than one, though, as you're likely to find that the second and third deep breaths come more easily than the first. Within just a few seconds, with only three deep breaths, you'll be able to detect where you are holding tension in your body. Is it in your abdomen, upper chest, shoulders, or buttocks? Maybe you can detect tension behind your eyes or even in your thighs. Wherever you noticed the tension, I'm willing to bet that it's where you hold it every day. When you release the tension in these muscles, you release the associated stress. If you can identify the source of the stress, you can address it.

When Should You Use Them?

Body breaks don't have to be long, so you can include them in your day much more often than you may think. Any time you notice you are having trouble concentrating, that your breathing has become shallow, or that there is stiffness in your body, is a good time for a body break. If you are unaccustomed to paying attention to your body signals, consider scheduling body breaks throughout the day. You can even use an alarm on your phone to remind you to check in with your body. To start, I recommend taking a body break once an hour. This will help you tune in to your "unique energy pattern"—the normal rhythms and cycles of your body—and gauge your current level of productive capacity. (I will go into this in more detail in Step 6.)

What Form Can They Take?

Body breaks can take many forms. If your work requires long periods of sitting, then you may want to move during your body breaks. If your work includes long periods of standing on your feet, you may want to take breaks that give you an opportunity to sit quietly for a few minutes. These are not hard and fast rules, though. Regardless of your physical position, body breaks serve to shift your focus away from the work at hand to your body and the world around you. Remember, their primary purpose is to assist you in remaining mindful and aware of your energy, and to reduce anxiety through perspective.

Review the menu of activities and select five that are most interesting to you. (The menu of suggested activities is by no means exhaustive. If something not listed comes to mind as you review the lists, go ahead and add it.) As always, trust your instincts and ignore any "should" thinking that could lead you astray. As one client responded when I told her that I'm not attracted to yoga, "Oh good. I thought I should be." I also have no affinity for prolonged "ohm-style" meditation, so I was relieved when Janet, the medical intuitive, told me that sitting in my backyard watching the birds fly in and out of our trees was an acceptable form of meditation. Again, one size does not fit all. Thank goodness!

If you worry that you will get lost in a body break, and not get back to work within a reasonable time, then use a timer to signal it's time to stop and go back to what you were doing. If you notice that you really don't have the energy to restart, I encourage you to pay attention and act accordingly. If you have any concerns about potential harm associated with any of these suggestions then, by all means, consult your health care advisor (doctor, etc.).

Menu of Body Breaks—Easy and Relaxing

What can you do lying down in bed or sitting on a sofa or chair?

- Arm, shoulder, leg, and neck stretches
- Deep breathing

(continued)

- Meditate
- Eat a healthy, delicious snack
- Take a 15–20 minute nap
- Chair dance to your favorite music (oh yes, you can!)
- Watch a favorite TV show, especially one that makes you laugh or smile
- Read or listen to an inspirational passage or chapter from a favorite book
- Talk on the phone with a good friend
- Work on a hobby for a few minutes
- Take a bath (although not in bed!)
- Play your favorite computer game
- Get down on the floor and play with your child, or your dog or cat
- Write in your journal (gratitude notes or success notes offer perspective in the face of worry)

What can you do outside, on a porch, or in the backyard?

- Almost everything listed in the previous section
- Watch the birds at play
- Inspect a flower or plant. Notice the details.
- Take pictures of people, plants or buildings in your area
- Walk around the block or your backyard (when my husband worked in an office he used to take a brisk walk around the block instead of heading to the nearest vending machine)
- Take a drive into town to get a snack or run a quick errand
- Water or weed your garden, or start one

The suggested activities on the following two lists will require a longer period of time than those on the two lists above. However, as I and others have discovered, the rewards of "extreme self-care" are well worth the time they take, especially if you enjoy them, too. If you are not familiar with any of the suggestions on this menu, and you notice you are curious about something, make note of it in your notebook and schedule time to do some research.

Menu of Body Breaks—Longer or More Rigorous

What can you do with the help of a professional trainer or healer?

- Any form of massage that is safe and relaxes you
- Craniosacral therapy
- Network spinal analysis (NSA)
- Physical therapy
- Reiki
- Chiropractic adjustments
- Yoga, in its many forms

What can you do as your strength and energy increase?

- Swimming
- Biking
- Power walking or jogging
- Hiking
- Hot yoga
- Weight training
- Golf

Select five body break activities from the lists above that you'd like to incorporate into your routine over the next two months. Then select two of them to start with in the coming week. If you need to learn more about any of the activities you've chosen, schedule the time to do your research now. If you need to talk to your doctor before starting a new activity, call him or her to set up a consultation, and prepare your questions. Decide how often you want to take each of the body breaks, and set reminders in your planning system until doing them becomes part of your routine. If making and keeping appointments with yourself doesn't come easily, be sure to read Step 6. Once you've finalized all these decisions, begin taking your body breaks as follows:

1. Start by incorporating each selected activity into your life for a week and make note of their impact in your comeback journal or record book.

2. Unless you don't like a new practice at all, continue with your chosen practices for at least two more weeks, as studies indicate that it takes at least 21 days to change your brain enough to effectively integrate a new habit[7] (to become, at the very least, consciously competent).
3. Review your results, make a new commitment to continue with the practices that are helping you remain unhurried and that are enjoyable. If you're ready, add another one from your initial list of 5.
4. Repeat as per above.

80% IS GOOD—UPDATING EXPECTATIONS

Life is not school. A+ doesn't mean "perfect with extra credit." At the end of your life, you will not regret your failure to be "perfect." You are much more likely to regret time not spent enjoying life with people you love. I think you already know this, but experience shows that as your symptoms stop presenting as an insurmountable barrier to productivity, you will feel pressured, once again, to put work before people and health, and to push beyond your limits. To prevent myself from giving in to that pressure, I adopted the 80% rule. I look at everything I feel I must do in one day, and remind myself that if only 80% gets done, life will still go on. I encourage you to adopt the same philosophy, especially if you are prone to project failure onto unfinished to-do lists.

I have slowed down to a virtual crawl—compared to many of my colleagues, anyway. People think I'm busy, but I am not. I am focused, and that is different. My daily task list is short and I have learned that I can work effectively on one significant project at a time. Yes, a goal of 80% is most certainly good enough. Here is how some of the people you've met in this book made similar adjustments:

- Upon returning to work, Joelle vowed she would not "rush to lunch" ever again.
- Bob and Peggy, the realtor and mortgage loan officer, respectively, returned to work committed to honor their values more than the cultural standards of their industry.

- C.J., the business coach and author, reduced her daily task list from fifteen to seven items, and stopped working at 5:00 PM even if she only accomplished six of them.
- Debbie, the scientist, gave herself permission to let go of a prestigious position in order to tend to her health and figure out what was really important to her.
- Susan, the speaker and professional coach, changed her business model in order to do more of the work that taps into her passion and skill set, and to reduce financial vulnerability in the future.
- Kelly, the missionary, let go of a life plan to do missionary work overseas in order to tend to his health. He continues to bend with life's changes as they are presented.
- Nedi, the musician and songwriter, reclaimed her dream to be a singer and songwriter, and teaches piano to young children in order to make ends meet.

These kinds of changes don't happen overnight, they happen over time. It takes courage and faith to adjust your expectations and redirect your life. Illness gives you a new perspective; it reveals courage you may not have known you had. 80% *is* good enough. Assuming that your goals are worth your time and effort, getting four things done out of every five you plan is a cause for celebration!

5 Things to Remember, Try, and Discard

5 Things to Remember

1. Focus on well-being
2. If you don't get it done today, it will be there tomorrow
3. Slow and steady might just win the race
4. 80% is good enough
5. Body breaks are good for business and your health

5 Things to Try

1. Do something that makes you feel at one with the world, like yoga or meditation, or even watching the birds outside your window
2. Eliminate one tortuous activity from your list of obligations
3. Cook something on the stove, from scratch
4. Implement two body breaks of your choosing this month
5. Keep a log for 1 to 2 weeks. Notice when you feel physically good, and when you feel tired. Do you detect any patterns?

5 Things to Discard

1. The worry habit
2. The rush to get back to work
3. Super-human perfection thinking
4. Productivity equals worthiness
5. Addiction to stress

Step 6:
Build Capacity, Organize for Success

*Balance is not better time management, but better
boundary management. Balance means making choices
and enjoying those choices.*

—BETSY JACOBSON

In Step 5, we concentrated on how to get your heart and mind to accept a slower rate of getting back to business. Step 6 is all about practically addressing the challenge of getting back to work, and creating a routine around work and self-care that will be adjustable as your health improves and your priorities change.

PLAN FOR UNCERTAINTY

Unless you work for a manufacturing company in an assembly line, your work-flow plan will not be neatly laid out for you. Even when the scope of your work is narrowly defined, any project you undertake will be comprised of a series of steps. The steps are not identical. Some of the steps will be interesting to you and easy to execute—and others won't be. These variances are individual and will impact the time required to finish a project.

Typically, productivity experts look at a project as a sequence of tasks, where the time required for each step is fairly uniform. While this method can work for establishing general guidelines, adding a human being to the equation introduces a variable. Variables are, by definition, less than absolutely predictable. Why does this matter? Because most people tend to underestimate the time needed and overestimate their "productive capacity" whenever any kind of variability is involved—even when the project they're working on is similar to one they've done in the past. When you take this approach, you suffer, your work suffers, and no one is very happy. However, there is a way to remedy the situation.

The first order of business is to establish a baseline of relative certainty. For example, if you are limited to working only four hours a day, it is not wise to fill your action plan with activities that are likely to require six hours to complete, nor is it wise to choose projects you anticipate will require the entire four hours. Both approaches fail to reflect anything approximating reality. The first approach sets you up to over-extend yourself. The second approach includes no room for contingencies or interruptions. To create more certainty in this four-hour-a-day scenario select tasks that, based on past experience, will consume no more than three-and-one-half hours. This builds in a small cushion for the unexpected. If you are able to finish the planned work in three hours, you can choose another small project that you can complete in about thirty minutes (see the end of this chapter for 30-minute task suggestions.). If you are having a "good day," and are able to continue working beyond the four hours you planned for, review your priorities and choose another project to start. You could argue that by starting out with a task list that would fill six hours, you won't have to stop and think to figure out what else to do if you can continue beyond four hours. Although this is true, it smells an awful lot like "business as usual," which is not viable approach at this time in your life.

Some people, like Kerry, a woman who gets debilitating migraine headaches about ten days each month, have an even more difficult time establishing a baseline of certainty. Her headaches are not only frequent, but also have no discernible pattern that will allow her to plan around them. She is as ambitious as any business owner I've ever met. Feeling frustrated with her inability to predict their arrival in her life, she asked for my help. She wanted to offer workshops via teleseminar. Knowing there was a strong chance that she would be overcome by a migraine at the time of the teleseminar, she was not sure how she could, in good conscience, schedule these kinds of events. We brainstormed solutions and alternative means for delivering her material, as follows:

- Instead of holding live teleseminars, she could pre-record her webinar programs.
- She could develop do-it-yourself multi-media programs that would include an ebook and/or a sequential email program.
- She could hire a Virtual Assistant with sufficient skills to moderate a workshop with her, or in her absence.
- She could find a business partner or form a strategic alliance with someone in her field, someone who could step in and take over if she could not conduct the workshop.
- She could tell program participants about her situation and give them advance notice of a potential need to reschedule.

Each of these options is less than optimal, with the last option on the list being the least favorable. It has the potential to create a lot of personal anxiety for Kerry. Furthermore, since she can't predict her migraine "schedule" she may have to reschedule an event more than once. However, it's also the reality of Kerry's situation, and these alternatives are certainly better than cancelling her workshops altogether.

Your unpredictable variables may be different from Kerry's, but they're no less disruptive. The more you understand them, the more you'll be able to work in harmony with them, decrease your stress, and increase your ability to accomplish your goals.

REDEFINE PRODUCTIVITY

In today's business world, billing clients by the hour and spending the entire day in the office is the default practice. However, it is a practice born in a different era, when manufacturing output was the primary basis for measuring productivity. The manufacturing model is no longer a fit for many different kinds of businesses, yet it remains the basis for most business practices. As Seth Godin wrote in his book, *Linchpin*, "You weren't born to be a cog in the giant industrial machine. You were trained to become a cog. [Furthermore], the rules were written just over two hundred years ago; they worked for a long time, but no longer. It might take you more than a few minutes to learn the new rules, but it's worth it." I dare say that your illness has given you an opportunity to reinvent yourself and rebuild your business or career under "new management."

Obviously, there are businesses for which people must be present in the office or on the factory floor for a specified period of time. However, I want to address the growing number of individuals working in or running companies that do not have a public brick and mortar location, and don't require a manufacturing operation to produce their products.

Typically, when people think about increasing personal productivity, they think about getting more done with fewer resources in the same amount of time. I say enough of that. We have inadvertently created a culture where living with the pressure of never-ending deadlines is normal. Ask someone how she is and you are likely to hear in reply, "crazy busy." Don't ask her what she is doing about it. She'll tell you there is nothing she can do—not this year, anyway.

There has been a movement in recent years towards recognizing the importance—and advantages—of building more flexible, people-friendly, results-oriented organizations. It is not an easy transition, though. Many owners, managers, and staff members remain strongly influenced by the old factory paradigm, do-more-in-less-time, which evolved into the corporate paradigm of keep-working-until-you-can't-anymore. Moving away from this mindset requires independent thinking; it requires that you question tradition and challenge the system.

Try to imagine this. What would your business life be like if you were to put the majority of your attention on just one or two important projects a day? Might it be easier to get more done? Would you feel more relaxed if you knew, with a high degree of confidence, that the projects you did not tackle today would be handled later in the week? Would your sense of well-being improve? If you are nodding your head, even tentatively, but have no idea how this is possible, keep reading.

THE SECRET IS IN THE SCHEDULE

"Your [Master Planning Schedule] helped me get some clarity on a struggle I've had for the last several months. What I realized is, while I don't want a J-O-B, I did miss some of the disciplines therein. Having the Master Planning Schedule is doing just as you said it would...bringing consciousness to my day. I know when I'm free, when I'm going to work and most importantly when I'm going to play. Freedom!!! I'm considerably closer to IDEAL than I was 24 hours ago and the reach doesn't seem so strenuous."

—TERRY A., CONSULTANT FOR NUTRISYSTEMS

Terry is just one of the many people who have successfully taken control of their work lives in absence of a corporate structure. Rather than working from a lengthy task list, Terry started orienting her task list and project plans around her "Master Planning Schedule" (MPS). The Master Planning Schedule is a map of your ideal week, a planning system that helps you stay focused on what is most important in your business or job, which enables you to use your best skills with increasing frequency, and accounts for your personal needs and priorities. By segmenting your business life into five to seven top-level areas of responsibility, and accounting for several other important factors I'll discuss in this chapter, you can improve your ability to identify where—and when—to put your attention to get the results you seek. Furthermore, because your available time and energy are factored into the plan, the plan will be realistic.

Figure 6.1 shows the first Master Planning Schedule I developed with a client in 2002. At the time, I was working with a mortgage broker who was feeling challenged by my suggestion that she group similar work tasks together in order to increase her effectiveness across the board. (See the Three Principles Behind the Master Planning Schedule on the next page for more information.) She bought into the principle but could not, for the life of her, see a way to ignore a ringing phone (a busy mortgage broker receives phone calls throughout the business day). However, answering client and prospect calls is not her only priority. Some of her work, such as entering client data into the loan application, is equally as important and requires a great deal of concentration, which is easily broken when she takes a call.

She asked me, straight out, "Joan, how can I dedicate two solid hours to data entry if my phone is always ringing?" In response I asked her, "Is your phone always ringing, or does it ring more frequently at specific times of the day and/or certain days of the week?" This was the pivotal question that she had never asked. After giving it some thought, she was able to see that it does not ring at the same rate throughout the day, but is heavier at specific times of the day and on certain days of the week, especially Monday mornings from 9:00 AM to noon. You can see, when you look at her Master Planning Schedule, that incoming calls are heaviest between 9:00 and 10:00 AM, and at the end of the day, so we blocked out those time slots accordingly. With this one insight, we were able to identify the best hours, including which day, to schedule her data entry work. Equally as important, on Monday mornings when the incoming call load was predictably higher, it was her job to answer the phone and make outgoing calls. It was not the right time to try to sit down and do data entry.

THREE PRINCIPLES OF THE MASTER PLANNING SCHEDULE

Principle 1: We are human beings, not human doings. Each of us experiences a natural ebb and flow to our productivity throughout the day, and no two of us are alike. I refer to the wave as your "Unique Energy Pattern." Furthermore, none of us were designed to be "on the go" for hours, days, and weeks on end. We need breaks, we need to stop and we need to have fun to restore our batteries each and every week. Once you understand your Unique Energy Pattern you can use this information to develop a work schedule that works with it instead of against it.

Principle 2: It's more productive to tackle similar activities in larger blocks of time[1] than to move rapidly from one activity to the next to the next and back again. The longer you can stay engaged in one kind of activity, the greater your momentum. You will feel more relaxed and the quality of your attention to the project or projects you're working on will be better. With this approach, procrastination will decrease and your ability to finish projects in a timely manner will increase.

Principle 3: Spend the majority of your time applying your strengths and talents to your most important business activities. This principle taps into the power of the Pareto Principle, often referred to as the 80/20 rule.[2] When you apply 80% of your time to the 20% of the business projects that make the greatest difference, you move into "flow." This is where you'll find your joy and your effectiveness.

Principle 1: Working with Your Unique Energy Pattern

No doubt you've heard the terms "morning person" and "night owl." These terms describe real preferences and natural rhythms of an individual throughout a 24-hour period. There's predictable consistency to your Unique Energy Pattern, which can only be detected once you stop pushing yourself to work against it.

	Mon	Tues	Wed	Thurs	Fri
	Laser	Support	Laser	Support/Free	Laser
7:00 AM					
8:00 AM	Church	Church	Church	Church	Church
9:00 AM		9–10 phone calls	9–10 phone calls	9–10 phone calls	Data input & wrap-up
10:00 AM	9–12 phone calls				
11:00 AM		Data entry	Constructive schmoozing	Data entry	Phone calls

FIGURE 6.1
Sample Master Planning Schedule

	Mon	Tues	Wed	Thurs	Fri
	Laser	**Support**	**Laser**	**Support/Free**	**Laser**
12:00 PM		Lunch	Lunch		Lunch
1:00 PM				Mary time	Phone calls
2:00 PM	Data input, analysis, etc.	File support	Client appointments		
3:00 PM					Data entry
4:00 PM	Phone calls	Phone calls	Phone calls		
5:00 PM	Wrap up phone calls	Wrap up phone calls	Wrap up phone calls	Wrap up phone calls	**Stop working**
6:00 PM	Dinner	Dinner	Dinner	Dinner	Dinner
7:00 PM			2 nights a week, meet with clients or networking.		

FIGURE 6.1 (Continued)

145

Your Unique Energy Pattern can be altered or disguised at various times in your life, and often is. Waking to an alarm clock will cause a disturbance in your patterns if the alarm goes off before you'd wake up on your own. Many report that their illness and associated medicines have impacted their energy patterns, either by keeping them awake at night, or creating a need for more sleep during the day. Teens, new parents, and midlife women—and some men—all experience disruptions and changes to their normal energy patterns, too.

Daylight hours appear to be the best time of day for the majority of people to be up and working. However, the nature of work is changing, and as we evolve, we may discover that more people do better work at differing times of the day than our historically rigid working lives have allowed for.

It is a shame when someone who admits that they naturally wake up at 7:00 or 8:00 AM is embarrassed to share this information with me. Their embarrassment stems from old, ingrained beliefs about success, such as "the early bird catches the worm." Accordingly, if you're not an early bird, you must be a loser. It's not only the "late" risers or the night-owls who feel uncomfortable about their "off" schedule. I know people who wake up at 4:00 or 5:00 AM, of their own accord. They, too, feel a little funny because they need to retire at 9:00 or 10:00 PM, precluding them from being one of the "cool people."

We have an interesting, often contradictory set of ideas about what it means to be cool and successful. They translate into "get up early and go to bed late." A client, the owner of a small, successful financial planning firm, realized that he believed that anyone who would leave the office at 5:00 PM was a "clock-watcher," aka a "loser." This only came to light when we were discussing the difficulty he was having getting up at 6:00 AM three or four days a week so that he could write for an hour before heading into work. This was the best time of day for writing, as he is, naturally, a morning person. Leaving work after 5:00 PM meant that everything was backed up into later evening hours, making it hard to get up earlier in the morning. By leaving the office around 5:00 PM, he would be able to spend the early evening hours with his wife and children, and still have some time later in the evening for his own endeavors before heading to bed. Loser no more!

I say it is time to release our robot-like conditioning and embrace our uniqueness. As I said before, I tend to wake up with the sun, which appears on the horizon at different times throughout the year, depending on its actual position and how we have set our clocks. I get up earlier in the summer and sleep later in the winter months. Sometimes I find myself awake in the middle of the night and get up and work. I don't fight any of it any more. I don't say I have insomnia, either.

A Successful Freelance Writer Relaxes into Her Unique Energy Pattern

Victoria, a freelance communications consultant and writer who works with established medical companies, responded with a sigh of relief when she was able to admit that she's really not ready to talk to people until 11:00 AM or 12:00 noon. As many people like her do, she often scheduled morning meetings with her clients at their request, without question. It never crossed her mind that doing this put her in front of her clients when she was not at her best, and that she had a choice about the matter. Once she was willing to consider changing her "internal company policies" around client meetings, we were able to map out a Master Planning Schedule that made more sense. Having already identified the important business activities that correlate with her preferred business roles, we incorporated her Unique Energy Pattern into her Master Planning Schedule. Instead of fighting her Unique Energy Pattern, she honored it.

It's not that Victoria didn't do anything before 11:00 AM. She started her workday at 9:00 AM, but she started it with lighter business activities appropriate to her disposition at that time of day.

She discovered, as have many others who prefer to work "off hours," that her best clients were able to work with her schedule without complaint. That is the key to all this. In order to orient your work life around a schedule that works for you, you have to be willing to test the system. You must be willing to take some risks with your business in order to build it in a way that works best for you. If you play it safe, and don't challenge your assumptions, your health and well-being will remain in the second position.

Do you know—or were you once—that grumpy employee who barely made it to work at 8:30 AM, miserable and dragging for the first few hours? Inside traditional business hours, this would have described Victoria. She would have been the person everyone complained about, wondering why she is so grouchy, and why it takes her until noon to become "human." To compensate, Victoria would probably drink a lot of caffeine-rich drinks in order to jump-start her energy. This is what happens when we operate as if everyone is the same.

The following questions will help you uncover your Unique Energy Pattern. While there is some overlap with a couple of the "perfect life" questions in Step 2, your answers to these questions will further refine your understanding of your ideal working schedule.

What Is Your Unique Energy Pattern?

- When do you have the most energy? For example, are you an early morning, mid-morning or an early afternoon person, or a night owl?
- When have you noticed that your energy drops in the day? After it drops, does it return? If so, for about how long?
- Can you detect your need for quiet vs. your need for activity? Can you correlate the need for each of these to specific times in the day?

(continued)

148

- When do you usually start your workday? Is this a good time for you, or do you wish you could start earlier/later?
- When do you need to stop working, either because of other obligations, or because you know you've exhausted your natural energy supply for the day?
- How much sleep do you need to be at your best?
- If it were completely up to you...
  - When would you wake up if not for an alarm, or some externally based obligation?
  - When would you go to sleep?
  - Do your answers correspond to the amount of sleep you said you need to be your best?
- Can you easily focus straight on through for hours at a time, without interruption, or do you work better in shorter bursts with intermittent breaks?

The best Master Planning Schedule accounts for your Unique Energy Pattern. After you have answered these questions, you can begin to think about when it's best to schedule your various business projects. Ideally, you want to set up a working schedule so that when your energy is highest you're working on your most important business projects, and when your energy is lowest you are doing tasks that require less brain power. We are quick to schedule appointments with clients, prospects, friends, medical personnel, etc., but very few people schedule appointments with their own projects. Quite frankly, failure to do so contributes to that feeling you get at the end of the day when you say something like, "I know I was busy, but I have no idea what I accomplished."

Principle 2: It's More Productive to Tackle Similar Activities in Larger Blocks of Time

Different types of tasks and projects require varying levels of energy and output. Administrative activities are qualitatively different than strategic planning activities. Data entry, or filing, utilizes a different set of skills and brain function than placing marketing calls or going out on appointments. Some business activities are task oriented, and others people oriented. (Remember the "hats" in step 3.)

Even if you can't organize your work schedule so that you are only working on one project for 2 or 3 hours straight, try to schedule your work so that energetically similar activities and projects are planned in the same 2 or 3 hour blocks of time. Operating with this degree of discipline may feel uncomfortable at first. If you are used to multi-tasking or working at a more hectic pace, staying with one project, or a narrowly defined set of tasks for a longer period of time, could ignite adrenaline withdrawal. Don't be surprised if you feel tired or restless as you experiment with this new way of operating. Don't let this "withdrawal" period fool you into believing you can't focus for longer periods of time without interruption.

If you can't stick with an activity—or energetically similar activities—for 2 hours, start out with shorter intervals. Try to stay with one activity for 30 minutes and gradually increase from there. Set a timer if it helps you keep on task. If you start feeling restless take a short body break, one that will help release tension without taking you off course. (I highly recommend staying away from email or social media when you are working on a meaty project, unless you use a timer to limit your time there. Those two activities can suck up time you really don't have.)

Principle 3: Apply Your Strengths and Talents Routinely to Your Most Important Business Activities

In Step 3, I asked you to think about the business hats (roles) that fit best so that you could improve your ability to put your time and attention towards the aspects of your business that are most rewarding, personally and financially. To help you make that determination, I included brief lists of the various business tasks that would be associated with those roles. I'd like you to refer back to the notes you made for that section as you think about how you'd design a Master Planning Schedule for your ideal week.

Once you assess your Unique Energy Pattern, and know which roles in your business or job are most satisfying and profitable, you can marry the information to draft your own Master Planning Schedule. It may be easier to do this if you own your own business. However, I have shared these techniques with the staff of several small businesses, as well as individuals who have hired me independently to help them improve their effectiveness and reduce their workload, and many have found it to be a useful tool.

IT Consultant Identifies His Essential Business Tasks

A computer consultant hired me to help him establish business practices that would increase his effectiveness during the workday so that he would be able to continue to grow at his targeted 20% annual growth rate while minimizing evening hours and weekend days spent on business tasks. He was highly motivated to make the necessary changes, due to the pending adoption of a newborn baby. To help him achieve his goals, he thought it a good time to hire his first employee, and wanted to figure out what role they should have in the business.

First, he identified his top three roles in the business, and then listed the various tasks and projects that come under each role. Using the same rating system that I introduced you to in Step 3, he gauged his level of interest, talent, and skill for each task using the "Love It," "Important," and "Ugh!" designations. Here is his list:

IT Consultant Evaluates Essential Business Tasks

Clients/Customer Service:

♥ Work with clients on-site and remotely
* Respond to support tickets
* Respond to emails
* Affiliate training programs for specific products and partnerships
⇓ Schedule appointments with clients (could also be classified under administration, below)

Online and Offline Marketing:

♥ Return/take phone calls from new clients, prospects
♥ Weekly blog post
♥ Update social media channels using Hoot Suite
♥ Visit local strategic partners to develop and nurture relationships
♥ Give presentations in local computer stores
♥ Meet with prospects on site for larger clients
♥ Weekly phone meeting with colleague in another state
* Review and post emails/responses on three targeted client base group lists
* Update all copy on website

Administration:

* Create estimates for new clients
⇓ Get all files together to send to bookkeeper for quarterly reports
⇓ Send out invoices
⇓ Manually enter all data from prior billing month to determine income

Going through this process clarified a few things for him. First, it highlighted the business priorities (which were primarily marketing related) that were important and fun for him, but were not making it onto his schedule with any regularity. Second, it was easy to see that much of what he enjoys is good for business. Third, it confirmed that he was justified in his recent decision to hire his first employee as soon as possible.

In light of the "ugh" notations next to most of the administrative tasks, you might think that he would hire someone to help with the administrative tasks first. However, with his goal of increasing annual revenue by 20% in mind, he decided to add a "junior" consultant first, someone who could handle the client-associated tasks that he marked with an *. He reasoned that in order to serve more clients, he needed someone to take care of the tasks associated with an anticipated increase in email requests and support tickets. Without such support, his growth goal would backfire on him. Using the Master Planning Schedule, he allocated the 2 to 3 hours he needed each week for regularly occurring administrative tasks, which he decided to handle for the time being.

Armed with this information, he hired his first associate and is on target with his revenue goal. His new daughter arrived earlier than expected. He was ready.

SOMETIMES YOU NEED A LITTLE PURPLE SNOW

My clients tell me that they love the idea of becoming more organized and focused, yet fear it at the same time. Creative people fear they'll lose their creative edge. People living with a chronic illness fear the unpredictability of their available energy. Parents and other care-takers never know when another person's priorities will take them away from their own. Allow me to lessen those fears with a little "purple snow."

The term "snow" (the color specification came later) was introduced into the Master Planning Schedule by Claudia, a new business owner in one of my first time management programs, and the mother of a 6-month-old son. Claudia was desperate to gain some control over her schedule, and wanted to understand how much time she really had to build a business and work with clients. After she drafted her Master Planning Schedule, she noticed increasing anxiety about her ability to stick to it in light of her son's unpredictable afternoon nap schedule. To address this, she told me that she needed to add "snow" to her plan. She called it "snow" instead of "free time" because she wanted to be clear about her intended use of that time, and she liked the feeling associated with snow. Good idea! During "snow" time, if her son was napping, she worked on a business project. If he wasn't napping, she tended to his needs. It seems like a simple mind-trick, but including "snow" in her weekly plan relieved the mental pressure she experienced when looking at a plan that didn't account for contingencies.

Another client, who was also feeling pressure about the appearance of an inflexible work plan, liked the idea of "snow" and decided to add "purple snow" to his calendar. (The Master Planning Schedule is usually created using different colors to represent different top-level activity categories. He chose lavender to represent "snow" in his calendar.) He was starting a second business and could be easily swept away by his greater interest in the new business project than in tasks associated with paid client work. Having established his baseline "financial set-point," he knew that he had to allocate at least 10 hours a week to billable client projects. "Purple snow," for him, represented the blocks of time that could be used for either billable hours or the new business project, depending on what else he needed to attend to that week. This strategy helped him stay true to his baseline financial commitment, while honoring his love for exploring new opportunities.

Recovery from a health crisis can be just as unpredictable as tending to the needs of a 6-month-old baby and as difficult to integrate as a new business project. Although these clients had different reasons for their "purple snow," you can benefit just as much as they did. By building flexibility into your schedule, you can account for any time your health might prevent you from finishing a specific project as planned.

A Human Resource Consultant Works Around Her Children's Schedules

Carlene, a human resource consultant with young children, stops working at around 3:00 PM most days, so she can pick up her children from school or daycare. From 3:30 PM until about 9:30 PM, her time and attention are devoted to family activities. She goes back to her home office two nights a week—this is a self-imposed limit—until 11:00 PM. Even though this schedule is not ideal, it is what works best right now. Since these later evening hours are lower energy times for her, she's decided that she will only select tasks from the following three business areas: reading and responding to email, conducting Internet research on topics relevant to her client work, and reviewing resumes on behalf of clients hiring new employees. They are tasks she enjoys and they don't tax her energy.

Carlene is not a fan of administrative work, especially billing, which she had previously been relegating to those later hours. Consequently, she felt even more tired in the evening—resistance is exhausting—and put those tasks off, anyway. At first, she thought it would be best to handle administration and billing on Friday mornings. Then she noticed that by Friday morning she was too tired to care, and another week would go by without doing them, thus slowing down receivables and increasing paper piles. Until she was ready to hire someone else to handle her administrative tasks, she decided to block out 2 hours a week for them, shortly after she starts work on Monday morning. There is another benefit to her revised approach. By bundling her administrative activities with planning her week on Monday morning, she starts the week from a strong position. Even better, she is freed from the mental weight—and self-recrimination—that she carried through the workweek, wondering if and when she would sit her rear end down and handle the administrative tasks. As we worked together to construct the best Master Planning Schedule for her, Carlene said, "I've been surprised by the feeling of liberation that I've had just since thinking about [scheduling] differently."

INVOKE THE POWER OF ONE

In *Work Less, Make More*, Jennifer White introduced a concept she called the "Power of Three" as an organizing principle for establishing priorities within a long list of tasks—the key being to choose the three most important tasks and focus our efforts on them. Of course, success with your chosen three projects or activities requires that you commit to those three things, above all else.

White explained the Power of Three as follows: "Anyone at any time can only put focus and energy behind three things. Three projects. Three big ideas. When you really put your passion behind three things, amazing results show up. Miraculous things. You're building momentum that allows you to get results faster than you do when you're juggling a multitude of things."[3]

I like the Power of Three for big-picture thinking (for example, what are my three most important roles in this business, or my three most important goals this month?) However, through observation and experimentation, I have begun to think that the "Power of One" is a more realistic model for establishing priorities on any given day. I am certainly more productive, and feel a greater sense of accomplishment, when I set my sights on completing one significant priority-oriented task each day. It's not that I don't do other things, but when it comes to moving an important project forward it is more realistic to decide which single project that will be. Furthermore, on days when my client schedule is full, that is my "one project" for the day.

This kind of focus can be challenging at first, but it is only your mind at play. The mind seems to want everything *now*. Even when you know what you most want to accomplish, your greater task will be to ignore your mind chatter. With practice—and later, success—your mind will be easier to ignore.

ESTABLISH YOUR FINANCIAL SET-POINT

I've talked a great deal about accounting for your health and your lifestyle preferences throughout this book. We've looked at how to reshape your business or career with these things in mind, and we've also touched upon the topic of money. The Master Planning Schedule can be used to bring all of these elements together. It is a good business planning tool for establishing your financial set-point. Here is how this works.

One year I decided that I wanted to double my annual revenue, so I reviewed my Master Planning Schedule to look at what I would need to change in order to achieve this goal. Initially, I thought that I might have to work more than my standard 35 hours a week, or reduce some of my "passion-project time." Neither option was particularly attractive. I decided to think about what would be required if I could accomplish this goal without changing the overall flow of my weekly work plan. In my ideal workweek, I work directly with clients on Tuesday, Wednesday, and Thursday, between the hours of 11:00 AM and 3:00 PM, which is equal to 9 hours a week, as I take a lunch break between 12:00 and 1:00 PM. I do, periodically, work with people after 3:00 PM, but I have learned that my energy is less reliable after 3 so they're not going to get the best from me. In my business, that's really important.

You might wonder, if I'm only working with clients 9 hours a week, what I am doing the other 26 hours. As a solo business owner and a writer, I include reading, writing, business development (marketing), and administrative activities in my Master Planning Schedule. As is often the case for all small business owners, not all my working hours are "billable" hours. This is true even when your revenue is not connected to billable time, or if you work for a company. The ratios change, depending on the nature of your business.

Back to the question at hand: I did want to double my revenue, so something had to change. Here were my options:

- Step up my marketing efforts to make sure that the 9 hours allocated to working with clients were, in fact, filled with client appointments. This was an obvious solution, but it's easy to overlook the obvious.
- Raise my rates by eliminating the lower-end coaching package, or keep my rates the same and increase the time allotted to client work by 3 to 4 hours a week.
- Keep the same client hours, but reduce the number of individual clients and add one group program in order to increase my revenue per hour of "client time."
- Add a new revenue stream entirely, such as on-site training and/or paid speaking engagements (this option had the greatest potential impact on my ideal working schedule).

By understanding the financial significance associated with the various options, I was able to make decisions about where to focus my efforts, what projects to work on, what to stop doing, etc. I was pleased to see that doubling my revenue was completely doable through minor adjustments to my overall weekly schedule plan. By using the Master Planning Schedule as a revenue planning tool, I have become more mindful of the projects and activities that are generating revenue and those that are not. It's also easier to say "no" to requests or opportunities that would keep me from doing the things I really need to work on. Furthermore, this exercise helped me identify tasks that must be done—but are not the best use of my time—and can be delegated.

IF YOU CAN'T DO IT ALL, WHAT CAN YOU DO?

Debbie, whom you met in earlier chapters, isn't ready to go back to work yet, but she has regained enough physical strength to begin to put structure into her routine and to tackle more projects. At the same time, she is aware of a tug-of-war within. As her strength and well-being started to come back, she has noticed the resurgence of old patterns of thought that threatened to regain control of her actions "fighting" with her newfound ability to remain relaxed, calm, and unperturbed. Sound familiar?

Debbie was already familiar with the Master Planning Schedule from our earlier work together, before she went out on disability leave. She asked to make use of it again, as she was beginning to feel much better and felt it would be important to her continuing recovery to be more productive. She remarked, "When I don't take a thoughtful approach to planning, I tend to default to the things that are familiar and comfortable, but may not be important." Additionally, she was not yet sure if she wanted to go back to her work as a scientist, or continue her education to become a science teacher, instead. Consequently, her MPS was not, at that stage, too overly structured, and we could use it as a general planning tool for her life as a whole, not just her work life.

To get started, we identified six top-level life categories for which she then listed various tasks and projects, as follows:

Physical Health: Exercise, medical appointments
Self-Care: Explore nature, read, sleep, meditate (it was important to Debbie that she distinguish between physical health and self-care commitments)

Home: Organize closets and garage, cleaning, cooking, shopping, gardening, cat care, house renovations, laundry

Relationships: Time with husband, communication with family, keep in touch with old friends and make new friends

Work/Study: Attend classes, homework, independent study projects, physics review, prepare for standardized exams, career exploration

Creative Outlets: Piano lessons, write poetry

Debbie was still experimenting with the reconstruction of her career and life "under new management." So, instead of blocking out the same time slots every week for the same tasks (as many clients choose to do), she used the lists above as a menu from which to select up to four tasks or projects a day. The selection of tasks from four of her six life categories signified her bottom-line commitment to productivity, and the menu aspect of her approach supported her intention to become better acquainted with what is most interesting and important to her. We came up with four filtering questions to help her make her selections, as follows:

- What will I do today to forward my physical health?
- What will I do today to forward my emotional health?
- What will I do today to forward my mental health?
- What will I do today to forward my spiritual health?

These were useful questions for Debbie, as they assured her that she was not going to ignore anything important. At the same time, she would not prematurely push herself into projects and commitments that would, in the end, not be healthy for her. After selecting her four daily projects, Debbie determined how much time she thought she would need to allocate to them that day, and used her paper planner to schedule them in the order she thought would be best.

A couple of years prior, Debbie started using a paper calendar system made by a company called Planner Pads®.[4] It's one of the very few paper planning systems I've found that comple-ments the Master Planning Schedule. Armed with her MPS, she could use the Planner Pad to identify and schedule her daily plan. Here's how it works: There are 3 horizontal sections. Across the top row, under the master heading "Weekly Lists of Activities by Categories," you can fill in your chosen work and/or life catego-ries. For each of the seven work/life categories, you then list up to ten specific tasks or projects you want to work on that week. (I recommend selecting no more than five.) You then drop down to the middle row, which has the days of the week listed hori-zontally. In this section, you select specific tasks (up to seven or eight) you want to accomplish on each given day. Underneath the middle section, at the bottom and across two pages, you can then schedule your outside appointments and internal project com-mitments. Debbie found this to be a very supportive planning system.

WHAT CAN YOU ACCOMPLISH IN 30 MINUTES?

I have shown you a variety of ways to use the MPS to slowly but surely build your productive capacity, and become more organ-ized around your top business and personal priorities. You may be like Debbie, who, as of this writing, is still putting more of her attention on self-discovery and recuperation than on rebuilding her career. You may be further along, and have the physical and men-tal strength to maintain a more traditional work schedule. Perhaps you're somewhere in between, and are only able to give 3 to 5 hours a day to your business or job.

Regardless of your circumstances, if you are susceptible to interruptions during working hours (who isn't?) you can still get quite a lot done. As long as you are able to concentrate on one task for 30 minutes at a time, much can be accomplished—even if you are limited in your ability to work. If you can concentrate for thirty minutes six times during the day, you're looking at 3 highly productive hours. The following are examples of what one person can do, from beginning to end, in a 30-minute time period:

What Can You Do in 30 Minutes?

- File a 1/2-inch stack of paper
- Compose two to three important emails
- Read and file or delete ten informative emails
- Delete obsolete files from your computer
- Outline or draft a blog post or article
- Review and edit one 500 word document (the typical length of a blog post or short article)
- Submit an article to one or two article list servers
- Research one idea
- Talk to a prospective client or networking contact
- Listen to or watch a recording of a webinar or teleseminar, or part thereof
- Meet with an employee or co-worker
- Develop your intended action plan for the week
- Pay bills or prepare a couple of invoices
- Interact with friends or fans on Facebook
- Read and respond to posts on your favorite LinkedIn group
- Tweet, re-tweet, and reply to your followers on Twitter
- Compose an Excel grid for tracking revenue
- Create 3–4 slides for a PowerPoint presentation

If you know what your priorities are for the day, you can select your 30-minute activities from this kind of menu. What would you add to the list of 30-minute tasks?

PRACTICE DISCERNMENT—KNOW WHAT'S NOT NEGOTIABLE

Any time you add a new project or opportunity to your life, you can use your Master Planning Schedule to understand the potential impact on your other priorities and projects. Realistically speaking, since there are only 24 hours in a day, any time you add a project or change your priorities, it will impact everything else and new choices will be required. A lot of people I have worked with find this fact frustrating at first, and then quite liberating. Previously, they felt uneasy about how hard it was to keep up with everything, or wanting to say "no" to something that didn't feel right to them. However, once they embraced the MPS, their confidence and sense of accomplishment increased so much, that it was easier to make these kinds of choices. As one client, a professional organizer, said, "I feel so much more relaxed now."

When a new opportunity or idea gets your attention, you have three options.

1. You can eliminate something else altogether
2. You can delegate a task or project that is important to you, but does not require your personal stamp, to open up the time for the new opportunity
3. You can reduce the time allocated for another project to make room for new commitment

The more you work with the Master Planning Schedule (or your equivalent) you may come to realize, like I did, that no matter what you might be interested in pursuing, some things in your life are not negotiable. (You may have uncovered some of these things when doing the exercises in Step 2 and earlier in this chapter.) In order to be a happy camper, any and all opportunities have to be assessed with them in mind. The following are my non-negotiable criteria. What are yours?

■ I need time each and every day to just think. If I don't have that on a regular basis, I become increasingly unhappy. I have noticed that when I go more than a couple of days without "thinking time," which is expressed through reading and writing, that I tend to wake up in the middle of the night. This is why I start working with clients after 11:00 AM, and keep Mondays completely open for writing, planning, and business development projects.

- I run out of steam between 3:00 and 5:00 PM on business days. This is the end of my productivity, at least as far as client work goes. I often take a 30-minute break after my last client, and then go back to my desk for another 60 to 90 minutes.
- I need 2 to 3 hours in the evening to wind down and do nothing of importance. Engagement with business thinking keeps me up past my ideal sleeping time, so I schedule evening business networking activities no more than two times a week. My family appreciates this too.
- I'm a second-thing-in-the-morning person. I'm at my best in the morning but not at 6:00 AM. I don't join networking groups or schedule speaking events that require an early commitment.
- I need to get to sleep by 11:30 PM for optimum sleeping. It's even better if I get in bed between 10:00 and 10:30 PM.
- I prefer two full weekend days off each week, although I am okay if I work 3–4 hours on Saturday or Sunday, if needed.

I speak of my non-negotiable parameters in absolute terms. Life is not absolute, though, and as I tell my clients, you can negotiate with your scheduling plan—with caution. As I and others have discovered, once you become aware of those times when you do make exceptions, you'll find that you can only do this up to a point. After you reach that point, you'll notice that you're back to where you were before: unhappy, overextended, and less effective. When I first started using this system, my non-negotiable commitments were a little different. You, too, may find that your non-negotiable parameters change over time.

Throughout the book, and in this chapter, I've shared stories of real people who have, through thoughtful review of their lives and business circumstances, reclaimed authority over their schedules. Whether healthy or ill, all were motivated by circumstances to figure out how they could restructure their work lives in a way that was both business- and life-friendly. When you set out to develop your own Master Planning Schedule for your ideal week, you may not know where to begin. I recommend you start by mapping out your weekly and daily non-negotiable commitments.

What Is Currently Non-Negotiable in Your Life?

- Do you have to get up by a specific hour in order to get children ready and out the door to school? Remember to include time to tend to your own needs.
- Do you want to wake up at a specific time because it's the best time to work on a personal project?
- Do you need to stop working by a certain hour in order to maintain your health?
- Do you have regular standing appointments with clients, customers, managers, or staff that cannot be changed, at least not now?
- Do you want to allocate time each and every week to people or projects that have nothing to do with work?
- How many full days off (no work, no business projects, no phone calls, etc.) do you need to remain relatively fresh and functional? Which day(s) would be best?

After you have mapped out the non-negotiable activities, you can start to fill in the rest of your MPS. The following questions will help you do so.

- What are the top two to four business roles that require your time and attention every week, if not every day?
- What specific tasks are associated with those roles, and must be scheduled on a regular basis?

- How much time do you think you need to dedicate to them every week (or every day)?
- When is it best to schedule them? (Remember to consider your Unique Energy Pattern when scheduling your various business priorities.)

Refer back to the sample Master Planning Schedule earlier in the chapter if you need a visual reminder of what it looks like once your regularly recurring priorities are mapped out.

MAKE AND KEEP APPOINTMENTS WITH YOURSELF

Your Master Planning Schedule serves you best when it reflects the way you want to live your life and run your business. When it's well designed, it will help you in those moments of choice when you receive an invitation, need to make a decision about scheduling appointments, or have to adjust to include a new circumstance, planned or unplanned. It's not your master and you're not expected to follow it to the letter of the design. When your priorities and circumstances change—and they will—you can update your Master Planning Schedule accordingly.

If you tend to "give your time away" to whatever and whoever comes your way, stop doing that. You can't afford it, and neither can your business. If you need to spend 2 hours a week working on administrative projects, decide when it is best to do such things (many people choose Friday morning) and put that in your Master Planning Schedule every week. If you need to keep up with industry standards, and that requires 90 solid minutes of reading, put that in your schedule.

Does this approach seem impossible? Then take yourself out of the equation and think of these various non-client or customer tasks as appointments that you are scheduling on behalf of your business. If you hired someone to handle these things, you would expect them to do what they said they would do, wouldn't you? Give your company as much of your great talent as you give your customers, family, and friends. Professional development, thinking, learning, and self-care are all legitimate aspects of a well-rounded, successful business person. If you can't do it all yourself—and there's a good chance you can't—go back to Step 4, "Recruit and Request—Ask for Help," and see if you can find someone to pick up the slack.

It takes courage to respond to requests without creating urgency at every turn. It's not necessarily comfortable to say, "I'll need a week to respond," or "I'm booked right now. I can schedule time for your project next month." I have heard all the arguments against setting strong boundaries around your top business priorities. They are always based in fear or lack of resources. Both are associated with "certain" threat over lost business or an uncomfortable conversation. Will you take the challenge, and return to business with new operating guidelines? I hope you will and I believe you can.

To be successful with this you have to be willing to do a few things:

- Believe it's worth your while.
- Be willing to challenge tradition.
- Remember that your Master Planning Schedule represents an ideal week. No week is ever ideal, but some come awfully close.

5 Things to Remember, Try, and Discard

5 Things to Remember

1. Your non-negotiable boundaries and commitments
2. You work better in flow with your Unique Energy Pattern
3. You are a human being, not a human "doing"
4. Employ your strengths and talents whenever possible
5. Plan for uncertainty

5 Things to Try

1. Put your personal/business projects in your schedule
2. Select just one high-priority project or goal each day
3. Account for "purple snow" in your schedule
4. Focus for at least 1 hour on something you care about every day
5. Schedule 30-minute activities if you are low on time or energy

5 Things to Discard

1. Working at all hours
2. Multi-tasking
3. The word "impossible"
4. Making yourself wrong for putting yourself first
5. Robot-like conformity

Epilogue: Write Your Own Comeback Story

Your time is limited, so don't waste it living someone else's life.
                                                        —STEVE JOBS

The people you've met in this book are just like you. They are ordinary human beings who are doing their best to live full, meaningful lives despite their circumstances. They have each, in their own way and on their own timeline, carved out new—often improved—ways of doing business and engaging with work. Like you, there are times when they have felt out of control and scared beyond belief. Like you, they are determined, strong-willed, and innovative. You have to be in order to continue working during and after a prolonged health crisis.

Now it's your turn. You've read the stories and done many of the exercises offered in the book. Regardless of the method(s) you used to take notes and craft your plans, you have at hand a manual from which to rebuild under "new management." Are you ready to take the next steps and write your own comeback story? Have you already started? I imagine so.

In addition to the gift of hope and insight, I expect you've started to develop the gift of trust and patience. Unless your health crisis is truly short-lived, with a clearly defined beginning, middle, and end, there will be times when you want to move forward and your body won't cooperate. This becomes especially frustrating as your energy and strength return. It's one thing to "surrender" when you have no choice. It's quite another thing to accommodate setbacks once longer periods of productivity have been experienced.

In Greek mythology, Sisyphus, a trickster known for his abilities to deceive gods and humans alike, was condemned for eternity to pushing a big, heavy boulder uphill. Although we forget the tale and the nature of his crimes, it's hard to forget the futility of pushing a boulder uphill. If you lose faith and push when you're not ready, you risk a similar fate. On the other hand, if you can become friends with "right timing," you'll not only ease your healing process, you're likely to discover the pure beauty of everyday life. It might help to picture yourself in a canoe, moving downstream with the current at your back. You still get to (have to) paddle to direct the course of your actions, but it's nothing like the energy required when you're paddling upstream.

As I was bringing this book to a close I was talking to a new client who, 4 years after back surgery, is preparing to get back to work. Prior to surgery, she worked for a well-known corporate consulting firm. At heart, she is an artist, one who happens to have strong analytical skills. After a great deal of self-reflection, she's decided to pursue a career in a more creative field, textile design. She is taking classes to learn her craft and pursuing unpaid internships. During one of our last meetings, she told me that she was having a lot of fun and felt guilty about it. She was uncomfortable because opportunities come easily to her, now and in the past.

I say that when you are on your "right" path your work shows it. When you are working in your "passion zone," you can't help but give it your all. It may not feel like work to you, but it is. I prefer to think that when you are aligned with yourself, life unfolds more easily.

So, when life feels hard and you're not achieving what you want as quickly as you want, it may only mean that either the timing isn't right or you need to change directions. Put your health and interests first, and life may become easier. Try this on for fun: Instead of feeling guilty when life unfolds with ease, embrace it. It could mean that you're exactly where you're supposed to be, doing exactly what you're supposed to do, even if that is convalescing.

CONNECT

It's common to feel isolated—and to isolate yourself—when you feel sick and weak. The need to withdraw your energy is a normal, preservation-oriented response to illness. However, withdrawal becomes a problem when it becomes a habit. Whatever distress caused you to withdraw has the potential to threaten your recovery if nursed for too long. Even if the size of your network decreases, it is important to stay connected with people you have cared about in your life, and who have cared about you.

You may recall that when Kelly accepted the wisdom of one doctor's advice—that if he wanted to continue to live and do his work, he'd have to stop doing ministry work overseas and head back home—Kelly immediately made contact with his network and set up fourteen interviews. That was only possible because Kelly stayed in contact and had earned the respect and trust of his professional peers. He could "bank" on his connections.

In the past, when I was so sick that I had to stay home and close to the bathroom, I didn't go out much at all and, even when I did it was on a very limited basis. At other times, when my symptoms were less disruptive and I felt mentally and physically well enough to attend, for example, a seminar I was interested in, if needed to I brought a light blanket and sat in back of the room. This helped me keep my body stabilized, and allowed me to be out with others, too. To increase my comfort, I told the seminar leader about my situation so that if I did need to leave the room I wouldn't feel the stress I would have felt if I had not divulged my situation. I had to give up "looking good" in order to participate and be with other people.

Following are four easy ways to connect. As always, choose whichever and how many are right for you.

1. *Listen*. You may not always have the energy to talk. That's okay. Turn your attention outward and ask a colleague or friend how *they're* doing. Remember that "being" is equally as valuable as "doing."

2. *Join.* Even if you can't get out and about as much as you have in the past, you can still participate in communities, either locally or online. In this day and age, it's much easier to connect with other people with similar interests. In the resource section you'll find a partial list of networks you can join, primarily online. There are so many more opportunities than I've listed. You can often access city and county directories of activities and groups in your area, too. Make a short list of criteria before you search: what topics are you interested in, do you want to meet online or in-person, and do you prefer to be an active or passive participant? Then start your search.

3. *Share.* Allow yourself to be vulnerable with other people. When you share yourself with others, it is a gift to them. Why? When you are authentic with others, they are likely to be more comfortable with you, too.

4. *Start a blog.* If you really want to swing out, start a blog to chronicle your thoughts and experiences. If connecting in this way appeals to you, it would be wise to think about the possible ramifications, especially if you're still in the job market. Many employers now search the Internet to see what candidates have put out online. If you are not willing to risk the potential loss of access to future opportunities, look for more private means of sharing yourself.

GIVE

One of the best ways to get your attention off your aches and pains is to help someone else. You can do that through your work, with family and friends, or through volunteer efforts. A few of the people I interviewed, and a couple of my clients, have found wonderful ways to give to others. (Some of them were already engaged in these efforts before they became ill.) One does prison ministry work at San Quentin (a federal maximum security prison in California), another is tutoring her niece and nephew, and another maintains a blog in support of sending girls in underdeveloped countries to school. Nedi is using her music to increase awareness of and to normalize people living with autism. I wrote this book—and the previous one—with an intention to encourage others on the same journey. Regardless of the instigating motivation, any act of giving is a sure sign that your illness need not stop you from living a meaningful life.

Giving comes in many forms, large and small. Play a game with a child. Invite someone to lunch in your home. (You don't even have to cook. You can order in.) Reach out to someone in a group you belong to: Invite a phone conversation or just send a quick note to tell them you appreciate them. Say hello to a neighbor. Send thank you notes by mail.

DISMANTLE THE SECRET SOCIETY

Since, according to census statistics, you're just one of over one hundred million people who are living with some kind of chronic condition, doesn't it stand to reason that the secrecy surrounding illness is disproportionate to reality? If I were not writing this book, and had not decided to specialize in coaching self-employed professionals reconstructing their businesses after a health setback, I would not have the conversations I now have. Whether I meet someone in a coffee shop or at a business meeting, because I answer the question, "what do you do?" with the above information, I often find out the "normal" person sitting next to me is also dealing with an illness. If they're not, someone close to them is.

Next time you worry about what someone will think if they find out you're not feeling well, think about this: Your neighbor or co-working may be suffering, too. If it seems appropriate to the conversation, and revelation will deepen a growing connection, why not let the cat out of the bag? Let's see if we can normalize a normal part of life.

MY MISSION

It is my hope that as technology makes it increasingly easy for people to work from anywhere in the world, that the barriers to doing meaningful work, even if on a limited schedule and from bed, will decrease significantly. I think improved access to healthcare and medical insurance will be essential ingredients for such a change. (The Patient Protection and Affordable Care Act [PPACA] of 2010 is a first step in that direction.) In addition, business owners, managers, and labor laws will have to change, too, placing greater importance on results produced than time spent at the office. Will you join me in the evolution? Visit http://www.JoanFriedlander.com for more information.

Resources

You can take the girl out of the bookstore, but you can't take the books away from the girl. A well-written book does three things: inspires, educates, and offers practical guidance you can use. Most of the books listed here have been on my shelf, and served as resources for me and (a few) for my clients.

Business, Health, and Productivity

- *The Big Enough Company: Creating a Business That Works for You* by Adelaide Lancaster and Amy Abrams (Portfolio Hardcover, 2011). This book was recommended to me by a former client, the mother of a grade-school daughter, who was having difficulty keeping up with the growth in demand for her services. In order to meet the demand she hired another service provider and then an assistant. She was perplexed by her increasing frustration and unhappiness. Through *The Big Enough Company*, she was encouraged to "right-size" her business so she could go back to doing more of the work she enjoyed, working directly with clients. She changed the business model to do more group work, and decided to stay smaller than she could have in light of demand. This is a good supplemental book for the work you did in Step 3: Back to Business Under "New Management."
- *The Creative Entrepreneur: A Visual Guidebook for Making Business Ideas Real* by Lisa Sonora Beam (Quarry Books, 2008). I chose this book to put together my "business plan" for 2012. Using a highly creative approach to planning (think colored pens, construction paper, and pictures from magazines), coupled

with important practical and tactical questions, the authors turn the normal drudgery of preparing a traditional business plan into a work of art. Imagery, coupled with key words, gives your subconscious mind access to your deepest wishes.

■ *Escape from Cubicle Nation* by Pamela Sims and Guy Kawasaki (Portfolio Hardcover, 2009). Even though this book was written for the new or thinking-about-it entrepreneur, it is a good resource for the experienced entrepreneur, too. It's been almost 12 years since I "escaped from cubicle nation" so I was delighted to discover that Sims' guidance is relevant to the entrepreneur in the middle of a major repositioning transition, too, or who just needs some practical and intelligent encouragement.

■ *Goal-free Living: How to Have the Life You Want NOW!* by Stephen M. Shapiro (Wiley, 2006). As a self-pronounced former "goal-aholic," Shapiro talks frankly about the potential tyranny of our goals, and the negative impact they can sometimes have on our experience of success and fulfillment. He doesn't completely dismiss the validity of goals, but he does put them in perspective. He prefers purpose and objectives, putting greater emphasis on being open to opportunities and whispered guidance in the moment than to pre-prescribed outcomes of goals and plans. Illness requires a more fluid relationship to goals and plans. It's hard to let go of years of training—to be successful you need a plan—and this book can help relieve some of that pressure.

■ *I Can't Be Sick: Contingency Planning for Really Small Businesses* by Mary K. Wilson (Juniper Gardens Press, United Kingdom, 2011—digital version available on the Kindle). This book is exactly what it sounds like: The author guides entrepreneurs through the process of creating a back-up plan for their business. Even though you're already in the midst of a crisis, it's never too late to begin future-planning. Wilson's book covers preparation for various scenarios, not just health crises.

■ *Steve Jobs* by Walter Isaacson (Simon & Schuster, 2011). This is the biography of perhaps one of the most well-known entrepreneurs of all time—who also spent a great deal of his career battling cancer. The book details how Jobs was able to realize his vision of Apple, Inc., while also chronicling the difficulties he went through with his disease.

- *The War of Art* by Steven Pressfield (Warner Books, 2003). Pressfield says that the closer you get to your passion and your purpose, the greater your resistance becomes. It seems backward, doesn't it? Shouldn't the obstacles and fears melt away once you stand face-to-face with your greatest dreams? No, apparently not. Resistance speaks in many voices: "That's stupid," "That's not possible," "I can't because," "What will they think of me if I do that?" "Who really cares about that?" and the like. Easy to read and a lot of fun, *The War of Art* will help you quiet the voices that keep you from pursuing what you hold dearest.

- *Work Less, Make More: Stop Working So Hard and Create the Life You Really Want* by Jennifer White (Wiley, 1999). White passed away in 2001 at the age of 33, suddenly and without warning. Nonetheless, *Work Less, Make More* remains relevant today. At a time when people are working hard and feeling frustrated and unfulfilled, this book encourages the reader—whether self-employed or working for a company—to take charge of their life and career. Easy to read, the 10-steps of the Work Less, Make More® program are smart, reasonable, and doable.

Finances

- *Estate Planning for People with a Chronic Condition or Illness* by Martin M. Shenkman, Esq. (Demos Health, 2009). Marty is a well-known speaker and author on estate and tax planning. In 2006 his wife, Patti, was diagnosed with Multiple Sclerosis (MS). "Surprised at how many of his professional colleagues were ignorant or just plain insensitive to the daily challenges facing those suffering from MS, Parkinson's, and other chronic illnesses," Shenkman wrote this book and started speaking to other planning professionals. In addition to more traditional end-of-life topics, he addresses questions regarding life insurance, living trusts, power of attorney, and when to work with a lawyer.

Marketing

- *Book Yourself Solid: The Fastest, Easiest, and Most Reliable System for Getting More Clients Than You Can Handle Even if You Hate Marketing and Selling* by Michael Port (Wiley, 2nd edition, 2010). Next to *Get Clients Now!*, Port's *Book Yourself Solid* is one of the best marketing books I've run across for service professionals (a good model for home-based business owners). I use his book with my clients whenever I am working with someone who doesn't like—or fears—marketing, who doesn't know what to say to people, or what marketing methods will work for them. Port has done an excellent job guiding business owners towards understanding their "who, what and why," the foundation for all marketing strategies.
- *Get Clients Now!* (GCN) by C.J. Hayden (Amacom, 2nd edition, 2006). GCN helped me tremendously when I started my coaching business. As a licensed facilitator since 2002, and a member of Hayden's internal team from 2003 to 2009, I taught this program to more than 400 independent business owners. Hayden demystifies marketing and, beyond that, gives you a structure for action around a specific 28-day business goal. Whether experienced or new to business, *Get Clients Now!* will elevate both the quality of your marketing efforts and your results.
- *The Jelly Effect: How to Make Your Communication Stick* by Andy Bounds (Capstone, 2010). *The Jelly Effect* is a good supplemental book to the other two marketing books listed here. Using a more structured approach than Port, he focuses on what he calls "the afters" to help readers get into the heart and mind of their prospects and clients. (The "afters" describe the experience your customers have while and after working with you. If you have a hard time talking about the benefits of your services or products,

this book will help.) *The Jelly Effect* has proven to be a useful supplemental book for business owners and sales professionals who are targeting larger businesses, too.

Self Recovery and Discovery

■ *Finding Your Own North Star: Claiming the Life You Were Meant to Live* by Martha Beck (Three Rivers Press, 2002). Martha Beck is a renowned author and life coach, and a regular contributor to *O* Magazine (Oprah). *Finding Your Own North Star* is just one of several well-known books, including *The Joy Diet* and her more recent book, *Finding Your Way in a Wild New World*. With humor and optimism, Beck takes you on a journey deep into yourself, helping you further articulate your ideal life. Once identified, she guides you from dreaming to planning to implementation. It's not an easy journey, but it is possible.

■ *Refuse to Choose: Use All of Your Interests, Passions, and Hobbies to Create the Life and Career of Your Dreams* by Barbara Sher (Rodale Books, 2007). *Refuse to Choose* is one of my favorite books, as Sher brilliantly addresses the reality of life as a "Scanner." Scanners are idea people, driven more by their need to learn, explore, launch, and create than those who are wired to be focused on a single job, career, or project from beginning to end. Not all Scanners are the same. Sher helps readers determine which of the 8 Scanners they most resemble, and then shares tips and strategies for each type so that they can embrace their true nature *and* be more effective and productive in their business or career. If you feel badly because you never seem to finish what you start, this book will change your life. Other similar books by Sher include *I Could Do Anything If I Only Knew What It Was* and her first, *Wishcraft*.

■ *Tough Transitions: Navigating Your Way through Difficult Times* by Elizabeth Harper Neeld, PhD (Bargain Book, paperback edition: Grand Central Publishing, September 13, 2006). In *Tough Transitions*, Dr. Neeld demystifies and illuminates the choices individuals will need to make in order to successfully navigate all kinds of transitions, from the more positive (such as a new baby) to the more difficult (including illness), through the four stages: Responding, Reviewing, Reorganizing, and Renewing.

- *The Way of Transition: Embracing Life's Most Difficult Moments* by William Bridges (Da Capo Press, 2001). Bridges' lifelong work has been devoted to a deep understanding of transitions and to helping others through them. When his first wife of 35 years died of cancer, however, he was thrown head-first into the kind of painful and confusing abyss he had known before only in theory. Filled with heart and compassion, *The Way of Transition* explains the three stages of transition (endings, the neutral zone, and beginnings), bringing normalcy to often confusing and disruptive experiences.

Career Discovery and Success

- *100 Conversations for Career Success: Learn to Tweet, Cold Call, and Network Your Way to Your Dream Job!* by Laura Labovich and Miriam Salpeter (Learning Express, LLC, September, 2012). Labovich and Salpeter are professional career coaches. This book helps job seekers manage their day-to-day search and professional networking in-person and online. Job seekers who need this book know they should reach out to business contacts and connect on social media, but don't know how. The book includes scripts and templates that teach you what to say.
- *Creating You & Co.* William Bridges (Da Capo Press, 1998). I've not personally read this book, but knowing the quality of Bridges' writing about navigating major life transitions, I put it on the list. Amazon says of this book, "Bridges shows true security comes not from clinging to a job, but from doing the work you're best at for the employers who need it. By learning that approach you can cement your value to your current employer, shape a new job for yourself, actually start a small company, or blaze your own path." I agree.

- *Do What You Are: Discover Your True Career Path through the Secrets of Personality Type* by Paul D. Tieger and Barbara Barron-Tieger (Little, Brown and Company; 4th revised edition, 2007). Based on the Myers-Briggs Type Indicator (MBTI) assessment, the Tiegers guide readers to understand suitable career options based on your "Type." Many books of this kind are hard to follow. When I used their self-assessment process to determine my type (INFJ), I found it comparatively easy. In addition to offering countless career options for your type (some will resonate and some won't) they discuss the gifts and drawbacks of your type, the critical criteria for job satisfaction, and share real stories of different career paths for people with your type.
- *Employment Issues and Multiple Sclerosis* by Phillip Rumrill and Steven Nissen (Demos Health, 2nd edition, 2008) covers quite a few questions that a patient with multiple sclerosis might have about his or her career. I have not read this book.
- *Get a Life without Sacrificing Your Career: How to Make More Time for What's Really Important* by Dianna Booher (McGraw-Hill, 1996; available from Amazon.com, used). Booher's easy-to-read book is filled with tips to help you be more efficient and productive, without undue stress. With only two or three pages per tip, you can flip through the book any time you want a little boost of inspiration and insight. Tips cover such topics as decision making, delegation, managing relationships, and simplifying your life.
- *Get Hired Now!* by C.J. Hayden and Frank Traditi (Bay Tree Publishing, 2006). Using the same action template for success presented in *Get Clients Now!*, Hayden and Traditi wrote a book to help people looking for a new job create a targeted 28-day action plan for the next phase in their search. In addition to the plan, itself, this book helps job seekers understand what really works to land the kind of job you seek, with top billing given to personal connections and networking.
- *How to Find the Work You Love* by Laurence Boldt (Penguin Books, Revised edition, 2004). I turned to this small, wisdom packed book, to help me answer the question that I was driven

to answer when things went awry in my career, "What do I really want to do with my life." Coupled with the book, *Do What You Are, How to Find the Work You Love*, it helped me access the inner guidance that often eluded me.

- *Social Networking for Career Success: Using Online Tools to Create a Personal Brand* by Miriam Salpeter (Learning Express, LLC, 2011). Per Amazon.com, this book shows you "how you can create an effective, compelling online presence; ... how social networking can propel your career; the ins and outs of social networking sites (LinkedIn, Twitter, Facebook, Quora, and many more), from the basics to the advanced features; tips for creating and maintaining a blog that will establish you as an expert in your field; and much more."
- *Women, Work, and Autoimmune Disease: Keep Working, Girlfriend!* by Rosaline Joffe, M.Ed., and Joan Friedlander (Demos Health, 2008). WWAAD covers the steps necessary to bounce back from being diagnosed with an autoimmune disease. The book offers hope and guidance for women in their career building years, managing the ups and downs of an autoimmune illness who want to continue to work. You'll read stories about real women who, with varying levels of success, were able to get back to work, and frank discussions about the issues and challenges that threaten to derail women, in particular (employer and societal expectations, inner beliefs, and family pressure).

Health and Wellness

- *Anatomy of the Spirit: The Seven Stages of Power and Healing* by Carolyn Myss (Three Rivers Press, 1997). This book may not be the right book for everyone. However, if you are willing to entertain the possibility that what ails you in your body contains a psychological and spiritual component (as Myss puts it, "your biography becomes your biology"), then I strongly recommend this book. The author blends diverse religious and spiritual beliefs—everything from the 7-tiered chakra system to the symbolic power of the

7 Christian Sacraments—into an engaging discussion of health and human anatomy. She manages to take heady material and anchor it in real-life issues through the experiences of real people.

- *Chronically Happy: Joyful Living in Spite of Chronic Illness* by Lori Hartwell (Poetic Media Press, 2002). "As a small child, [Hartwell's] kidneys became permanently damaged after she ingested *E. coli* bacteria. At age 12, her kidneys shut down completely. Over the next decade, Hartwell underwent dialysis, countless surgeries, and two failed kidney transplants. Her third transplant, in 1990, was a success." Hartwell shares her own story of triumph and emphasizes the importance of attitude on your ability to live a successful, joy-filled life, regardless of personal circumstances. Included in her guidance are frank suggestions about "what to do about work," the importance of connections and "how to fight pain until you win."

- *A Delicate Balance: Living Successfully with Chronic Illness* by Susan Milstrey Wells (Da Capo Press, 2000). Wells gives the reader a good sense of how to rebuild a normal existence after a life-changing diagnosis. *A Delicate Balance* covers a wide range of topics—from seeking treatment to dealing with personal relationships—and is geared toward someone who has recently been diagnosed.

- *I Didn't Sign Up for This! 7 Strategies for Dealing with Difficulty in Difficult Times* by Sandra A. Crowe (Two Harbors Press, 2012). The day she moved into her new home, Crowe became extremely ill. Her new home literally made her sick and she struggled with a debilitating chemical sensitivity illness. She had to abandon her new home and for years searched for a diagnosis and treatment. She couldn't stay anywhere for long and often slept in her car. Topics include: how to design and shift your emotions no matter what, where and how to change expectations so your mood does too.

- *Who Says I Can't? A Two-Time Cancer-Surviving Amputee and Entrepreneur Who Fought Back, Survived and Thrived* by Jothy Rosenberg (Bascom Hill, 2010). This is the story of a man diagnosed with cancer as a teenager, who then went on to become a champion athlete and manager of a start-up company.

CONNECT—INTERNET-BASED COMMUNITY NETWORKS

Clearly, during the times you are housebound, if you have enough energy and are inclined to connect with people on the Internet, any of the primary social media platforms can be utilized to do so. On the other hand, if your time and energy are limited, you may want to be careful about how much time you devote to connecting on-line. As always, it's a personal choice, one that is well served by periodic assessment. Ask yourself this: Does your engagement convert to a worthwhile reward, either for your business or your sense of personal well-being?

Each of the top three platforms—as of this writing: Facebook, LinkedIn, and Twitter—has a slightly different feel and use. Furthermore, in addition to connecting with friends and former colleagues, you can find groups—or start one—where people gather around specific topics and professions. The platforms and groups are continuously changing. Use the following brief descriptions to gauge your interest and spark ideas.

Note of caution: the more communities you join, the more email you will potentially receive. You can minimize the impact of incoming emails from these communities by changing default settings on each platform so that you only receive what you want to receive. Personally, I receive no group post notifications from Facebook (except my own), and stopped all group notifications from LinkedIn. If you want to minimize the incoming notifications, yet engage with some frequency, decide how much time each day, or how many days a week, you want to check these group postings and schedule the time in your Master Planning Schedule and on your calendar.

General

- *Facebook:* Facebook is currently "the friend" place. Used by individuals and businesses with equal zest, you can pick and choose your own parameters for engagement. Some people use Facebook to keep up with family and friends, and nothing more. Others use it to engage with both business and personal networks. If you are a business owner or want to create a community around a cause, you can create two separate identities, one personal and one cause or business oriented. For the latter, as of this writing, you can create either a fan or group page. (The look and feel of Facebook evolve frequently and the rules keep changing.) http://www.facebook.com

- *LinkedIn:* LinkedIn remains the premier platform for business professionals. If you use Facebook for maintaining personal connections, you might use LinkedIn to establish and maintain professional or business connections. I encourage you, especially if you have been isolated for a while, to use this platform as a means to stay current with your professional network and to participate in groups that are either geographically or occupationally centric. There are also LinkedIn groups devoted to specific health topics, although the few I've joined seem to be spattered with people who offer services or products for these groups. As a result, some posts are clearly more marketing- and sales-oriented than support-oriented.

- *Twitter:* Twitter is both a personal and business platform and the preferred social media home for many celebrities, who can collect thousands and millions of followers. (In 2011, the top celebrity had over 27 million followers.) Unlike LinkedIn and Facebook, it is not a permission-based platform. Twitter is very fast paced, so the more followers you have and the more people you follow, the easier it will be to get "lost in the crowd." You can talk to people in your Twitter network, but it's harder to follow the trail of communications than on Facebook. If you use Twitter as a platform to connect or promote your brand or business, I would suggest that you plan to post at least 2 "tweets" a day, Monday through Friday if not every day. http://www.twitter.com

Biznik, Quora, Google-Plus and Pinterest are gaining in use, but I have not used them so I will not comment.

Health and Illness Communities

The following communities and sites represent just a sliver of those that have been formed in recent years. Some are private groups, ensuring a higher degree of confidentiality, and others are public groups. By all means, do your own research to look for resources that would support you. You can search for health or disease groups on Facebook and LinkedIn, and search for blog sites that discuss an area of specific interest to you.

On Facebook—Health and Disease

Because website addresses (URLs) change and pages close, I'm not including page addresses. Do a search on any of these page names—or similar terms—and you'll find them and many more.

- *Cyclic Cushings Disease Network:* Run by Pat Gurnick, a psychotherapist in Colorado who knows what it takes to navigate the impact of a dramatic illness, offers counsel through this page, helpful to people with Cyclic Cushing's Disease, applicable to all people on the healing journey.
- *Dr. Isaac Eliaz:* Dr. Eliaz is an integrative, holistic doctor, with a focus on treating cancer and chronic illnesses. As a researcher, product formulator, and clinical practitioner, he is dedicated to empowering people in overcoming disease and finding true health.
- *IBD or Inflammatory Bowel Disease:* Love this page for the unbashed bathroom humor depicting situations anyone with an IBD (Ulcerative Colitis or Crohn's Disease) can relate to.
- *Tigerlily Foundation:* "Non-profit organization dedicated to educate, advocate for, empower & provide hands-on services & support to young women, before, during & after breast cancer."
- *Thriving with MS:* "Your home for inspiration, conversation, and resources to live well while living with MS. We empower you with small, daily choices for living pain free and full of life."

ON FACEBOOK—SMALL BUSINESS AND CAREER

Note: All of the Facebook page owners listed below host a corresponding standard website, too.

- *Awesome Women's Hub:* A popular page in my Facebook network, the Awesome Women's Hub, run by Robin Rice, offers a dynamic, supportive community for women in business. Her tag line is "sharing awesome women with the world."
- *Barbara Sher:* Anything Barbara Sher writes is apt to inspire. She's a huge advocate for living your right life, and for crafting careers that tap into your unique talents. Per her Facebook fan page, "It is her mission to save as many geniuses as she can before she leaves this planet." (Hint: Everyone is a genius. The trick is to figure out yours.)
- *HubSpot:* Everything inbound marketing. They put out an excellent series of free ebooks on a variety of timely topics relevant to small business marketing today.
- *OnStartUps:* Practical advice for start-up entrepreneurs. Fun, information-packed page.

BLOGS AND WEBSITES

- *Care Pages:* One of my former clients used this site to stay connected to her personal network throughout her cancer treatment. It is an online diary platform. You select the people to invite and post anything you wish whenever you wish. The people who accept your invitation receive notice of your posts by email, and sign in to comment (and encourage!). A great resource from which to "let your hair" down with people you trust, and no one else. The site also hosts discussion forums on a variety of health-related topics. http://www.carepages.com
- *ChronicBabe:* A fun, lively site for women living well with chronic illness. "ChronicBabe offers hundreds of resources designed to help you keep on being a Babe, even with chronic illness." http://www.chronicbabe.com/

187

- *Hope Café:* Launched in late 2011 by Donna Sales, a therapist in Canada, Hope Café offers regular posts and life stories that inspire and encourage people facing any number of challenges. http://www.hopecafe.net
- *JoanFriedlander.com:* This is my own site. I write posts about the opportunities and challenges pertinent to those getting back to business after a health setback. Interviews, guest posts, program information, workshops and a resource section round out offerings on this site. http://www.JoanFriedlander.com
- *Keep Working, Girlfriend:* Even though Rosalind Joffe and I are no longer posting to this blog, if you are living with one of the 63 autoimmune illnesses and need guidance and support for continuing to work, look through archived posts on Keep Working, Girlfriend. http://www.keepworkinggirlfriend.com
- *Meetup.com:* Meetup.com is a good resource when you want to connect with people in your area. Topics of common interest span a wide range, from social to hobbies to business. Once on the main site, just enter your geographical area and keywords that pertain to your interests to get started. http://www.meetup.com
- *RV4The Cause—Helping those living with chronic illness:* In my search for financial planning resources for people living with chronic illness, I came across this site, run by Marty Shenkman and his wife, Patti. Even though this site is primarily aimed to educate other planners on the financial issues facing people with chronic illness, their mission includes consumers, as follows: "Empower those living with chronic illness and their loved ones to better plan their estates and finances through informing their advisers, free seminars for consumers," and the distribution of their book on the same topic (see Books, Finances). http://www.rv4thecause.org
- *TheGirlfriendGroup (TGG):* TGG is a free membership-based community and was founded by Vanessa Maddox in August, 2009, just a couple of months after her sister, Valerie, passed away. Says Vanessa: "We were extremely close and her death affected me to the depths of my soul. Valerie loved her girlfriends; they were like her family." TheGirlfriendGroup is both a professional

and social networking site, which mission is to help women in all aspects of life. http://thegirlfriendgroup.ning.com/

- *Treatment Diaries:* "Treatment Diaries is a social network for those living with illness, newly diagnosed or caring for someone with a medical condition." You can join this private community and select specific illness categories in which to commune with others about what ails you. If you need a safe place to vent, and feel inclined to offer encouragement and support, too, this would be a good choice. http://www.treatmentdiaries.com

OUTSOURCING—GET HELP WHEN YOU NEED IT

Virtual Assistants: If you have hesitated to hire help because you don't have the resources, or the amount of work typically associated with hiring someone either part time or full time, it would be worth your while to look into hiring a virtual assistant. They are "virtual" because they work in their own home office with their own equipment. They usually work for several people (owners or individuals), so they are considered independent contractors. They often specialize in the kind of assistance they offer, everything from desktop publishing to social media management to bookkeeping. The number of resources for searching has grown tremendously in the past ten years. When I hired my first assistant, there were only a couple of official training schools so searching was easier. You will increase your hiring success if you are patient, clear about your needs and requirements (including geographical location of your assistant(s), and take the time to screen, interview, and train. The following are a few websites for virtual assistant training programs from which you can learn more about the profession and search for help.

- *Assistant Match:* http://www.assistantmatch.com
- *AssistU:* One of the original training schools for virtual assistants. I posted my first request for help to find my first virtual assistant. https://www.assistu.com

- *Expert VA Training:* http://www.expertvatraining.com
- *VA Classroom:* http://www.vaclassroom.com/

The following are aggregate sites on which to search for freelance workers in a huge variety of professions around the world.

- *eLance:* http://www.elance.com
- *Guru.com:* http://www.guru.com/index.aspx
- *Odesk:* https://odesk.com

PRODUCTIVITY SOFTWARE

- *Evernote:* I was introduced to Evernote during an interview with a business owner for this book. When doctor and self-care appointments required her to be out of her office with some frequency, Evernote significantly increased her efficiency. It works across multiple platforms (on your primary computer, smart phone, and even the Nook). If you're taking notes for a project, or come upon a website page you want to refer back to, whichever platform you're using at the time, you can clip and/or create a note in Evernote right then and there. Furthermore, you can create different folders for different areas of your life so it's easier to categorize your notes. I use the free version.
- *Dropbox:* Though similar to Evernote, it is more limited in use. I have used it as a temporary file back-up system. I also used Dropbox to share book files with my editor so that she could grab new chapters as I finished them, and upload edited versions when she was done. To keep my other files private, I simply created a new folder for the book's files and invited her to see only the files in that folder. Syncing between your computer and the cloud is instantaneous. Dropbox creates a level of security that sending files through email does not. I use the free version.
- *Dragon Naturally Speaking* Voice-recognition software: This relatively low-cost software has been helping people for whom typing is difficult, or who prefer to talk instead of write.

Now on their 12th edition, the speech-recognition capabilities have improved significantly. The more you use it, the better it works. I use the home edition. It works in Word and in Outlook, and for Internet navigation (although that's a little harder to figure out.)

"LOW" TECH EQUIPMENT AND ERGONOMIC ASSISTANCE

In business, we tend to focus on technology solutions that make our lives easier. "Low" tech assistance can supply much-needed support for your body when pain or weakness accompanies your illness or injury. If you have medical insurance, check to see if occupational therapy and/or "medical durable equipment" are covered. If so, find out what is covered, as well as what the limitations and referral requirements are.

Following are a few resources to help jump-start your thinking about what you might use that would ease strain and/or rebuild strength in a way that is appropriate to your current level of physical health. Typically the purview of occupational and physical therapists—and a new field, adaptive technical professionals—if your health care professional has not yet suggested these kinds of solutions (mine never did), you may want to consult with them before purchasing any equipment. It will save you time and money.

■ *AliMed:* Medical and ergonomic products for healthcare, business, and home. AliMed carries over 70,000 of the most frequently needed ergonomic products. "From wrist rests to mousing supports, seating, and industrial aids, AliMed is your complete ergonomic resource." The website is organized into specific areas of need so you can narrow down your search. Clearly, the website is targeting professionals and healthcare specialists. As a potential end-user, a site like this can help you think about getting assistance that you may never have considered. http:// www.alimed.com

■ *Patterson Medical:* Similar to AliMed, Patterson Medical is another resource for physical assistance and rehabilitation equipment, offering a wide range of products. For example, under "Rehab supplies," you'll find a variety of products that help restore balance and with total body conditioning, information about exercise bands, balls, and weights, and even aquatic rehabilitation equipment. In addition to products, the site includes an index of sales representatives and consultants you can talk to in 18 metropolitan areas around the United States. http://www.pattersonmedical.com

■ *Worksite Health and Safety Consultants:* Dr. Naomi Abrams and her team have made it their business to improve the working conditions at the office, either a home office or traditional office. Whether you're working from bed, or sitting at your desk, good equipment, and correct posture and movement will help you be more productive and feel good, too. Check out their website for informative blog posts, articles, books, and to inquire about their consulting services. http://www.worksitehealthandsafety.com

Bibliography and Notes

PROLOGUE

1. White, Jennifer. *Work Less, Make More: Stop Working So Hard and Create the Life You Really Want!* New York: John Wiley and Sons, 1999.
2. Hayden, C. J. *Get Clients Now!: A 28-Day Marketing Program for Professionals, Consultants and Coaches*, 2nd Ed. New York: Amacom Books, 2006.

INTRODUCTION

1. Drake, Daniel. "Perfectly Happy: The New Science of Measuring Happiness has Transformed Self-Help." Boston.com, Globe Newspaper Company. March 9, 2010. Excerpted from dissertation by Samuel Bagenstos and Margo Schlanger in "Disabilities and the Average Happiness Index." (2007) Accessed July 4, 2012, http://www.boston.com/bostonglobe/ideas/articles/2009/05/10/perfectly_happy/?page=3 "Samuel Bagenstos and Margo Schlanger, law professors at Washington University in St. Louis, co-wrote a law review article in 2007 suggesting that the emphasis on lost enjoyment of life in jury awards actually makes it harder for the plaintiff to recover. Better, they argue, to focus remedies not on the lost happiness, which in many cases will take care of itself, but on specific lost capabilities, and on mitigating their effects through rehabilitation. And to the extent that disabilities do cause unhappiness, it's often from social factors like isolation and discrimination—so paying people off just for their disability may be counterproductive, since it can leave the real causes of unhappiness unaddressed." http://www.boston.com/bostonglobe/ideas/articles/2009/05/10/perfectly_happy/?page=3
2. Institute for Health and Aging, University of California, San Francisco. "Chronic Care in America: A 21st Century Challenge," a study of the Robert Wood Johnson Foundation & Partnership for Solutions: Johns Hopkins University, Baltimore, MD, for the Robert Wood Johnson Foundation (September 2004 Update). "Chronic Conditions: Making the Case for Ongoing Care." By 2020, about 157 million Americans will be afflicted by chronic illnesses, according to the U.S. Department of Health and Human Services. Accessed November, 2009. http://www.rwjf.org/files/publications/other/ChronicCareinAmerica.pdf

3. Institute for Health and Aging, University of California, San Francisco. "Chronic Care in America: A 21st Century Challenge."
4. U.S. Census Bureau. "Non-Employer Statistics." Non-employer businesses are described as those "businesses without paid employees that are subject to federal income tax." Accessed July 5, 2012, http://www.census.gov/econ/nonemployer/index.html
5. Joffe, Rosalind, MEd, and Joan, Friedlander. *Women, Work, and Autoimmune Disease: Keep Working, Girlfriend!* New York: Demos Health, 2008.

CHAPTER 1

1. Eckhart, Tolle. "You Are Not Your Illness." Excerpt from a free webinar series entitled *A New Earth: Awakening to Your Life's Purpose*, Eckhart Tolle. Produced by Oprah Winfrey and Eckhart Tolle on YouTube via Skype, Accessed March 23, 2010, http://www.youtube.com/watch?v=poSnBO3AWZg.
2. Neeld, Dr. Elizabeth Harper. *Tough Transitions*. New York: Warner Books, Hatchette Book Group, USA, 2005. Chapter 1, Responding, 33–93.

CHAPTER 2

1. Pressman, Sarah, "KU Research Finds Human Emotions Hold Sway Over Physical Health Around the World." KU (Kansas University) News Release. March 4, 2009. Accessed July 5, 2012, http://www.news.ku.edu/2009/march/4/emotion.shtml.
2. Peterson, C., and M. Seligman. *Character Strengths and Virtues: A handbook and classification*. Oxford, U.K: Oxford University Press, 2004.
3. Hayden, C. J. *Get Clients Now! A 28-Day Marketing Program for Professionals, Consultants, and Coaches*, 2nd Ed. New York: Amacom, 2006. 83–87.

CHAPTER 3

1. Amable, Teresa, and Steven, Kramer. "Do Happier People Work Harder?" *New York Times*, September 3, 2011. Accessed April 7, 2012, http://www.nytimes.com/2011/09/04/opinion/sunday/do-happier-people-work-harder.html
2. *The Jelly Effect: How to Make Your Communication Stick* by Andy Bounds (Capstone, 2010). Bounds points to what he calls "the afters" to help readers get into the heart and mind of their prospects and clients. The "afters" describe the experience your customers have during and after hiring you or using your products.
3. Hayden, C. J. "Entrepreneur on a Mission: What's your business model?" February 8, 2012. Accessed April 16, 2012, http://www.cjhayden.com/entrepreneurship/whats-your-business-model/. Excerpted with the author's permission.

CHAPTER 4

1. Guilt. *Dictionary.com's 21st Century Lexicon*. Dictionary.com, LLC. Accessed May 22, 2012, http://dictionary.reference.com/browse/guilt.
2. The U.S. Equal Opportunity Employment Commission (EEOC). "The ADA: Your Employment Rights as an Individual With a Disability." Last modified on March 21, 2005. Accessed July 6, 2012, http://www.eeoc.gov/facts/ada18. html
3. Walsh, Karen Vandermaas, email message to author, July 3, 2012.
4. U.S. Equal Opportunity Employment Commission. "Notice Concerning The Americans With Disabilities Act (ADA) Amendments Act of 2008." Accessed July 6, 2012, http://www.eeoc.gov/laws/statutes/adaaa_notice.cfm.
5. U.S. Equal Opportunity Employment Commission. "Questions and Answers for Small Businesses: The Final Rule Implementing the ADA Amendment Act of 2008." Accessed July 6, 2012, http://www.eeoc.gov/laws/regulations/ adaaa_qa_small_business.cfm. The ADA Amendments Act of 2008 (ADAAA) was enacted on September 25, 2008, and became effective on January 1, 2009.
6. "Questions and Answers for Small Businesses: The Final Rule Implementing the ADA Amendment Act of 2008." http://www.eeoc.gov/laws/regulations/ adaaa_qa_small_business.cfm.

CHAPTER 5

1. Hart, Archibald D. PhD. 1995. *The Hidden Link between Adrenaline and Stress*. Nashville, TN: Thomas Nelson.
2. Aronson, Dina, MS, RD. "Cortisol – Its Role in Stress, Inflammation, and Indications for Diet Therapy." Today's Dietitian, Vol. 11, No. 11, P. 38, November, 2009. Accessed: May 10, 2012, http://www.todaysdietitian.com/ newarchives/111609p38.shtml
3. Wilson, Dr. James L. "Adrenal Function in Autoimmune Conditions." Accessed May 10, 2012, http://www.adrenalfatigue.org/autoimmune-disease.
4. LeMaistre, Dr. JoAnn. "Coping with Chronic Illness," adapted from the book, *After the Diagnosis*. (CO: *Alpine Guild, Inc*. 1985, 1993, and 1999 by JoAnn LeMaistre.) Accessed May 10, 2012, http://www.alpineguild.com/ COPING%20WITH%20CHRONIC%20ILLNESS.html
5. Norton, David. "The 7 Essential Factors in Forecasting the Length of Homeopathic Treatment of Chronic Diseases." Accessed June 4, 2012, http:// www.homeopathyzone.com/blog/article/7-factors-forecasting-length-homeopathic-treatment-chronic-diseases#4
6. Epstein, Donald Dr. Network Spinal Analysis™ (NSA) also known as Network Chiropractic, was founded and developed by Dr. Donald Epstein. For more information visit http://www.donaldepstein.com/ (Accessed June 4, 2012).

7. Dean, Jeremy. "How Long to Form a Habit?" PsyBlog. Published: 21 September 2009. Accessed July 8, 2012, http://www.spring.org.uk/2009/09/how-long-to-form-a-habit.php. Jeremy Dean is a researcher at University College London. To his point, research studies reveal that the actual time required before a new practice becomes easy and routine varies, depending on the nature of the practice and your attitude towards it.

CHAPTER 6

1. White, Jennifer. *Work Less, Make More: Stop Working So Hard and Create the Life You Really Want!* New York: John Wiley and Sons, 1999. I first learned about time blocking through White's book. She is not the only one to have pointed to this strategy as a means to increase effectiveness and reduce stress. Others include well-known authors, Julie Morgenstern and Dan Sullivan.
2. Pareto principle. Dictionary.com. *Dictionary.com's 21st Century Lexicon.* Dictionary.com, LLC. Accessed July 05, 2012, http://dictionary.reference.com/browse/pareto principle
3. White, Jennifer. *Work Less, Make More: Stop Working So Hard and Create the Life You Really Want!* 69–70.
4. To learn more about Planner Pads®, visit https://plannerpads.com/concept.asp.

Index